MEDICAL PLAN FORENSICS

MEDICAL PLAN FORENSICS
EXAMINING THE EVIDENCE

F. RANDALL CHILDERS, JR., CFC, DABFE

Copyright © 2024 by F. Randall Childers, Jr., CFC, DABFE.

Library of Congress Control Number: 2024907886
ISBN: Softcover 979-8-3694-1988-5
 eBook 979-8-3694-1987-8

All rights reserved. No part of this book may be reproduced or transmitted in any form or by any means, electronic or mechanical, including photocopying, recording, or by any information storage and retrieval system, without permission in writing from the copyright owner.

Any people depicted in stock imagery provided by Getty Images are models, and such images are being used for illustrative purposes only.
Certain stock imagery © Getty Images.

Print information available on the last page.

Rev. date: 04/30/2024

To order additional copies of this book, contact:
Xlibris
844-714-8691
www.Xlibris.com
Orders@Xlibris.com
858338

Thanks to my wife Cindy, my family for the encouragement on writing this book. My friend Sandy Ringer a Business and HR Consultant, Business Visions and friend for many years in the review of this book.

CONTENTS

Introduction xiii
    Establishing Your Team xv
    Code of Conduct xv
  Fiduciary Duty / Responisbilities..xvi
  The Consolidated Appropriations Act, 2021 xix

Types of Group Health Plans 1
    Fully Insured Plans 1
    Spaggregate / Fully Funded Self Funded Health Plans 2
    Self Funded Plans with Stoploss 2
    Fully Self Funded Plans 3
Matrix of the Plan 4
  Traditional Matrix for a Self Funded Plan................................4
  New Matrix for a Self Funded Plan 5
  Self Funded Vs. Fully Insured Plan..7
Anatomy of a Medical Plan 13
Stoploss - Risk Management 18
  What is medical Stoploss coverage?..18
  Who is the insured?..18
  What is the role of the plan document? 19
  How is loss defined? 20
    Specific Advancement 21
    Accommodation...22
    Terminal Liability Option (TLO) 28
    Defining a Claim Payment 33
Pharmacy Benefit Management (PBM) 43
Parties / Vendors to the Plan 49
  Plan Sponsor 49
  TPA / ASO Vendor 50

Stoploss Vendor..51
MGU Vendor..52
Insurance Agency / Agent Vendor......................................52
Consulting Firm / Consultant Vendor...............................53
Managed Care Vendor...55
Aggregator Vendor 55
PPO Vendor..56
PBM Vendor...56
PBM Auditing Vendor 57
Example 57
    Search Results Agent / Broker / Consultant 59
    Search Results Fidelity Security Life Insurance Company ..62
    Result AM Best Search 63
    Search Result Continuing Education..................................65

Information Request 68
    Plan Sponsor 69
    Contracted Administrator 70
    Banking Information Request 71
    License and E&O Requests..72
    Sample Letter Contracted Administrator.......................73
        Documents..73
        Reports...73
    Agent, Broker or Consultant 74
        Sample Letter to Insurance Agent......................................76
        Prescription Benefit Manager (PBM)................................78
        Sample Letter PBM Company...79
    PBM Auditing Company 80
        Sample Letter PBM Auditing Company...........................81
    MGU / Stoploss Carrier 82
    Aggregator...83
    Managed Care 84
    PPO 84
    Dissection Fees 84
    Administrator Compensation Disclosure.......................86
        Contracted Administration Fees:..86
        *Compensation Paid From Contracted Administrative Fees*86
    Disclosure of UR/PreCert/CM/DM/Wellness Plan 88

Contracted PBM and Administrator	95
Contracted Stoploss and Administrator	96
Stoploss Carrier and Underwriter:	96
Agent, Broker or Consultant of Record:	97
Forensic Decision Mapping	100
Stoploss Reimbursements	103
PBM Provider	105
PBM Auditing	109
Plan Sponsor	112
Contracted Administrator	115
Aggregator	119
Managed Care	122
Accounting	124
Accounting and Accounts	127
Timeline Documentation	129
Types of Account Structures	131
Contract Administrator Owns Account	131
Accounting	139
Bank Accounts	140
Hard Fraud	144
Soft Fraud	144
Bank Account Analytics	145
Health Plan Deposits	145
Required vs Actual Deposits	146
Census by participation category	147
Vendor Premium and Fees	148
Medical Claim Refund	150
Medical Plan Detail Report	166
Census Count by Month	168
Plan Cost Structure	168
Summarized Monthly Detail Report	169
Aggregate Report	171
IBNR Report	174
Specific Stoploss Report	176
Laser Analysis Report	177
Stoploss Specific Reimbursement Report	178
Aggregate Reimbursement Report	180

   Aggregate Minimum Attachment Report 181
   Deposit Report..183
   PBM Rebate Report..186
Fraud in Self Funded Medical Plans 187
  Hard Fraud 188
  Soft Fraud 188
  Documents and Agreements..189
  Vendor Fraud 191
   Modifying the Quote..193
   Hospitalist Scenario Two (Actual Case)............................200
   Fraud and Eye Doctors (Actual Case)...............................204
Money Laundering...206
  Organized Crime Defined 207
  Placement..208
  Layering 209
  Integration 209
IBNR and IRBNP 219
  FORENSIC ANALYSIS AND REPORT 220
  IRBNP..220
   Overview...220
   First Level..223
   Second Level 226
  Process 231
   Data Extraction 231
  Stoploss Contract 234
   Specific 234
   Aggregate 234
   Analysis 235
  Data Analytics...236
   2014 Plan Year 236
   Prescription Claims 238
   Summary 2014..239
  2013 Plan Year 239
  2012 Plan Year 241
   Aggregate Stoploss 244
  Administration Agreement 245
  Agreement important provisions 246

Stoploss Agreement 261
Agreement important provisions 261
Pharmacy Agreements Analysis 263
   OBJECTIVE 263
   INFORMATION REQUEST 264
      AGREEMENTS / CONTRACTS............................... 264
      DATA 264
   CPA MASTER PROGRAM AGREEMENT 265
   Summary of ABDC / PSAO 268
      Questions on PSAO / ABDC 269
   Computer CompanyRx System Agreement 270
   PBM Agreements 274
   Recommendations 275
1099 Issue 276
Contracted Administrator Issue 280
      PRIVILEGED AND CONFIDENTIAL
          SETTLEMENT 290

Acronyms Used in this Book 293
Bibliography 295

Introduction

This book is designed to provide the investigative tools and insight in dissecting a Medical Plan on a micro level.

The investigative tools are utilized for the dissection of Self Funded Medical Plans and provides the applications for dissecting Fully Insured Medical Plans. Fully insured plans are owned by the insurance company. Self funded plans with or without Stoploss are owned by the plan sponsor.

It is important when utilizing the investigative tools that the Forensic Examiner remain completely objective in making an accurate determination of the facts involved and the presentation of the facts in a written report. Subjective interpretations and personal opinions must be held back and utilization of objective facts should be the road map utilized in the investigative process.

In forensics, one issue leads to the validation or invalidation by other supporting data and agreements. Through the comparative analytics and the deeper dive into forensics the objective facts are revealed. Contained within the pages of this book is the process of gathering the facts, utilizing tools to validate or invalidate the information, providing the Forensic Practitioner with the processes in a methodical and precise structure to investigate the information and the presentation of the objective findings.

When presenting the report, be sure to have validated findings upon presenting the work and report. Depending on someone other than yourself or the team for compilation of the analytics can provide problems if they are not qualified. Even if you have received the reports from a plan source, you must do the work to present the fact of findings. There may be differences in what you are presented and the actual objective data compiled in the analytics. Utilize the comparative analytics to show and document and the differences. In other words "Trust but verify".

It is recommended to read the book: ***Forensics of a Medical Plan - Dissecting Health Benefits on a Company Level*** to get insight and an overview of the various components of the Architectural Vendors to the medical plan. In addition, the practitioner should go through a qualified certification program such as the Certified Forensic Consultant (CFC) program to understand how to navigate within the legal system, writing objective reports, contracting with hiring entities, conflicts of interest and other issues.

This book will contain some case studies with all of the identities changed as an example of how the investigative tools are utilized.

The tools and insight provided will allow the Forensic Practitioner to follow the evidence and provide the objective facts. Forensics is a base for getting to the truth.

Forensics is not for just finding the criminal elements but to offer solutions based on the findings. In the professional practice of forensics it is not one's job to define guilt or innocence but to present the objective facts to the hiring entity and allow the legal professionals to determine the basis of guilt or innocence based on the objective facts.

Establishing Your Team

Bringing together a team which has specific expertise is vital to the analysis and presentation of the objective facts. The team should consist of:

- Legal which has expertise in health plans,
- Pharmacist which has expertise in Prescription Benefit Management (PBM) for analysis of prescription claims, contracts and fraud detection,
- Underwriter for Stoploss contracts,
- Aggregator for networks, repricing, negotiations, Managed Care Organization with expertise in pre certification, case management,
- Third Party Administrator (TPA) for claims analytics, processing, Health Care claims analysis for health care claims for fraud detection,
- Actuary specific to Medical Plans,
- Forensic Accountant.

In my practice, I prefer that each of these entities have the Certified Forensic Consultant (CFC) designation or similar certification for their specialties.

Code of Conduct

Principles of Professional Practice

ACFEI and its members are to remain completely objective and use their ability to serve justice by making an accurate determination of the facts involved.

ACFEI members are not advocates for one side or the other. Members should not intentionally withhold or omit any findings or opinions discovered during a forensic examination that would cause the facts to be misinterpreted or distorted.

ACFEI members should not misrepresent or overstate their credentials, education, training, experience, or membership status.

ACFEI members are expected to refrain from any conduct that would be adverse to the best interest and purpose of ACFEI. Members are to be forever vigilant of the importance of their role and to conduct themselves only in the most ethical and professional manner at all times.

Source: http://www.acfei.com/about_acfei/principles/#sthash.QydvGxqt.dpuf

Fiduciary Duty / Responisbilities

When providing a group health plan can be challenging as well as rewarding. The employees that participate in the group health plan, their beneficiaries (dependents) as well as the employer benefit when the group health plan is put in place. Additionally, administering a group health plan as well as managing the assets require actions which have specific responsibilities.

Plan sponsors / employers must understand some very basic rules, especially the Employee Retirement Income Security Act known as ERISA. The plan sponsors / employer must meet a set of standards of conduct for those who manage the employee benefit plans and the assets of the plans as they are called fiduciaries. The ERISA covered group health plan is an employment based plan which provides medical care coverage, including hospitalization, sickness, prescription drugs, vision or dental. These benefits can be provided utilizing funds in a trust, purchasing insurance or self-funding benefits from the employers general assets. some key elements of a plan include:

- A written plan that describes the benefit structure and provides guidance for the day-to-day operations;
- A trust to hold the plan's assets;
- A recordkeeping system to track contributions and benefit payments, maintain participant and beneficiary information as well as accurately prepare the reporting documents; and
- Documents to provide plan information to participating employees and the government.

Many times employers often hire outside professionals such as third party service provides - Third Party Administrator, or, use an internal human resources department to manage some or all of the plan's day-to-day operations. There may be one or more officials with discretion over the plan which are the plan's fiduciaries.

A person using discretion in the administeering and managing a plan or controlling the assets of a plan is a fiduciary to the extent of that discretion or control. A fiduciary status is based on the functions performed for the plan, not just a person's title. Employers who sponsor fully or partially self-funded group health plans excercise some discretionary control over the plan's operation. The plan can identify the fiduciary by the ofice they hold or specifically by name or some plans may use an administrative committee or the company's board of directors.

The plan's fiduciaries will normally include the plan administrators, trustees, investment managers, all individuals excercising discretion in the administration of the plan, all members of a plan's administrative committee, if one exists, as well as those who select committee officials. Attorney's, accountants, and actuaries are generally not considered fiduciaries when they act in their professional capacities. Additionally, a third-party administrator, recordkeeper, or utilization reviewer who perform ministerial tasks are not a fiduciary; however, this can change if they exercise discretion in deciding a participant's eligibility for benefits. Those entities or individuals who exercise discretion or control over the plan are considered fiduciaries.

Based on the above information, it is important for the fiduciary to understand each part of the plan, cost, compensation, vendors to the plan, to make sure they and the plan are operating in the best interest of the members to the plan and their beneficiaries. Forensic review as well as tha analytics can provide the fiduciary the proper objective information regarding the plan as well as recommedations for the operation of the plan. The forensic review will provide fiduciaries information which is important for the responsibilities and are subject to standards of conduct due to acting on behalf of the group health plan participants and their beneficiaries. Those area include:

- Acting solely in the interest of plan participants and their beneficiaries and with the exclusive purpose of providing benefits to them;
- Carrying out their duties prudently;
- Following the plan documents (unless incosistent with ERISA)
- Holding plan assets, if the plan has any, in trust; and
- Paying only reasonable plan expenses.

The duty to act prudently is one of a fiduciary's central responsibilities under ERISA. This requires expertise in a variety of areas. A fiduciary who lacks the expertise will want to hire someone with the professional knowledge to carry out those functions. Prudence focuses on the process for making fiduciary decisions, so a fiduciary should document those decisions and the basis for those decisions. As an example, when hiring a plan service provider, TPA, PBM, Network, UR-Precert-Large Case Management-disease management, Stop-loss (MGU's) and others, the fiduciary may want to survey a number of possible providers, asking for the same information and providing the same expected requirements. The fiduciary can then document the process and make a meaningfule comparison and selection.

Source: https://www.dol.gov/sites/dolgov/files/ebsa/about-ebsa/our-activities/resource-center/publications/understanding-your-fiduciary-responsibilities-under-a-group-health-plan.pdf

The Consolidated Appropriations Act, 2021

The CAA introduced new compensation regulations under the preexisting No Surprises Act which will directly affect agents, brokers and consultants. Agents, brokers and consultants as well as subcontractors will now be required to disclose their compensation to plan fiduciaries. This new regulation went into effect on December 27, 2021, and will impact contracts and aggreements entered into or renewed on that date of after.

Source: https://www.benefitnews.com/advisers/opinion/how-the-consolidated-appropriations-act-could-lead-to-lawsuits

The forensic examiner will utilize the various forms, algorythms and analytics as provided in this book as a guide to provide the disclosed as well as non-disclosed compensation made to the vendors of the plan which include but are not limited to TPA, PBM, Network, UR-Precert-Large Case Management-disease management, Stop-loss (MGU's), Agents, Brokers and Consultants.

Types of Group Health Plans

The party requesting the Forensic Examination due to an issue that has arisen may or may not have the knowledge of the type of plan or the relationships of the vendors to the plan. It is the responsibility of the Forensic Examiner to understand the type of plan and the matrix of the plan in educating the party requesting the examination / investigation.

The information described below should be considered as a review of the knowledge the examiner has as it relates to the various types of plans.

We will discuss the four basic structures and the two matrixes as well as a review the chart differentiating the Self Funded Medical Plan and the Fully Insured Medical Plan.

There are Four Basic Structures for Group Health Benefit Plans. There may be different terminology used in describing the types of Health Plans / Medical Plans. However, the descriptions should remain relatively the same.

Fully Insured Plans

These Plans are offered by insurance companies and are traditionally available for organizations of 2 or more employees. The Plan Sponsor pays a set premium each month and the insurance company keeps the profits and risks. The rates are normally set based on the experience of the insurance company and the profits they need to generate for business operations and their shareholders. There is minimal flexibility in the design of these plans as they are determined by the State and the designs submitted for approval by the insurance company. The insurance company **owns** these plans and the Plan Sponsor is a participant.

Spaggregate / Fully Funded Self Funded Health Plans

This is a hybrid structure that allows a progression from a Fully Insured Plan to a Partially Self Funded Plan also known as a self funded plan with Stoploss protection. This is considered a fully funded plan. This plan has the ability to retain funds for the plan sponsor based on good experience for the plan year. It is important to note the retentions will be minimal due to the increased cost in the stoploss program associated with these plans. The plans are normally available for Employers with 25 or more employees participating in their medical plans and some organizations will make this type of program available down to 10 participating employees.

Self Funded Plans with Stoploss

These plans allow more flexibility than those of the Fully Insured and Spaggregate Plans. This plan has some additional risk over the Fully Insured and Spaggregate

Plans, but has a much greater potential in retention of funds and controlling renewal cost. This structure utilizes a specific and aggregate Stoploss for risk management of the plan. Typically, these structures will provide Specific Stoploss Advancement and the option to have aggregate accommodation in protecting the risk of the plan. There is a much better basis for getting good rates and in instances of good experience having a static or reduced cost for renewal years. These plans are normally available for employers with 25 or more employees participating in their medical plans.

Fully Self Funded Plans

There is **no** protection on these programs and the plan sponsor assumes all liability for claims. This does give the highest basis for retaining funds unused to pay claims as well as flexibility. This type of medical plan structure is for very large employers normally with a minimum of 5000 employees participating.

It is important to understand the type of health benefit plan structure the organization is utilizing. The Spaggregate Plan, Self Funded with Stoploss and the Fully Self Funded Plans fall under ERISA if it is a private entity or public entity. These same structures exist for a government entity but are usually categorized as Non-ERISA Plans.

The focus of this book will be based on the types of **Self Funded Health Plans**.

Matrix of the Plan

The very fact the company has a health benefit plan which is self funded does not suggest there is an understanding of the architecture of the vendors to the plan. There are two different architectures for the plan. Each of the components are the same. However, the entity that controls the agreements with the vendors is very different. In the information below we will look at the two different matrix's for the plan. Understanding the difference in these structures can provide insight to the Forensic Investigation in the relationship of the vendors to the medical plan. Each of the Matrix's below will provide the foundation for the Forensic Decision Mapping in the relationships of the vendors.

Traditional Matrix for a Self Funded Plan

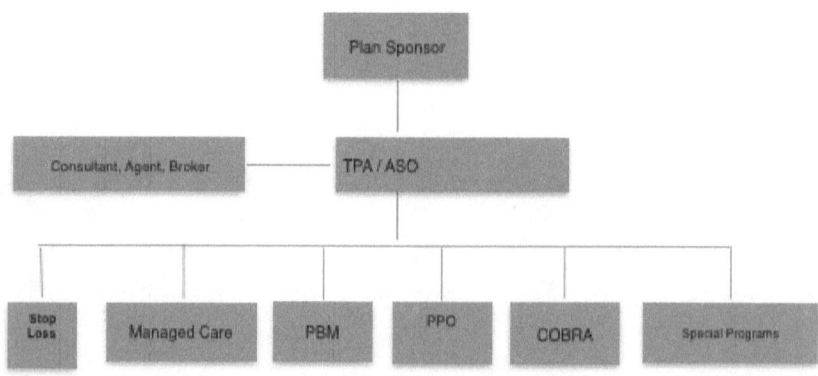

With the Traditional Matrix the plan sponsor is contracting with the Contracted Administrator, either an independent TPA (Third Part Administrator) or an insurance company ASO (Administrative Service Only), for the administration of the health benefit plan. The TPA/ASO is directly contracting with the various vendors to the plan. The Agent / Broker / Consultant is normally receiving compensation by contracting with the TPA / ASO witch includes either fees, commissions or both. The compensation for the TPA / ASO as well as the Agent / Broker / Consultant may not be fully disclosed in this model due to arrangements with the various vendors. The TPA / ASO may have transparent or non transparent agreements which provides compensation. This compensation may be considered non-disclosed (non-transparent) or may be disclosed (transparent) to the Plan Sponsor on the compensation received from the vendors to the plan.

The Plan Sponsor with the traditional matrix, the TPA / ASO is controlling the Plan Vendors. (This matrix is the same typically used in a fully insured health benefit plan). This is considered a bundled approach. Many TPAs / ASOs will not accommodate new vendors introduced by the Plan Sponsor specific to their plan as it may interrupt a cash flow to the TPA / ASO from their bundled agreements.

New Matrix for a Self Funded Plan

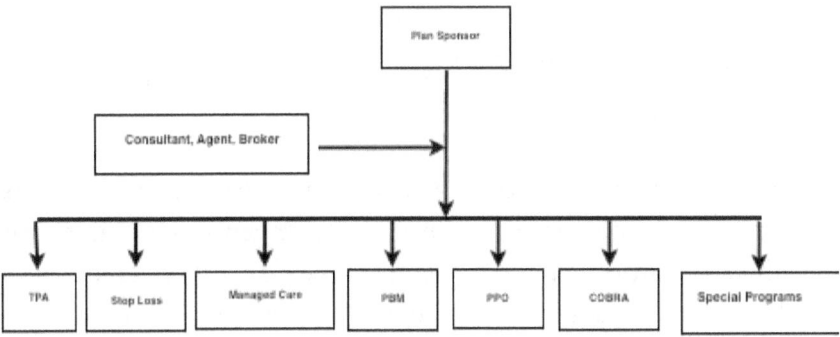

This is the basic structured matrix for a Self Funded Medical Plan. The difference is how each of these components are handled in the vendor architecture and contracting by the Plan Sponsor. In the Traditional Matrix, the Contracted Administrator (TPA/ASO) would have presented each of these components as part of their "Quote" to the Plan Sponsor. The Plan Sponsor would only see the numbers in the quote and not what is going on behind the scene. What is not shown in the quote is the additional income via fees, markups, commissions, rebates etc. that are possibly being received by the TPA / ASO / Agent / Broker / Consultant from the vendors of the Plan.

This New Matrix is the new structure for employer sponsored Self Funded Medical Plans. The Plan Sponsor contracts with each entity directly giving total control over the health benefit plan. The Agent / Broker / Consultant is normally the conduit in the architecture of the structure bringing the various partners / vendor architecture to the Plan Sponsor. This structure allows for total transparency in compensation with each partner.

The vendors in this model must perform, especially the TPA / ASO as they are now a provider to the plan and not controlling the partners / vendors for their financial gain. The TPA/ASO only receives their disclosed fees for services provided. All Stoploss and vendor agreements are net of commissions allowing a pure rate on the Stoploss without mark up.

The PBM, Prescription Benefit Manager, is contracted to pay 100% of the eligible rebates to the Plan.

This structure allows for accountability and transparency in all aspects of the plan. If a vendor is not performing then a new vendor can be put in without jeopardizing the architecture in the plan. All vendors utilized are chosen for their ability to help control cost and provide outstanding service to the Plan Sponsor and the participants in the plan.

In principle, the New Matrix should have fully transparent agreements. However, it is important for the Forensic Examiner to review the agreements and provide the same investigative savvy as would be done on the Traditional Matrix. **Do not assume anything, always investigate. The findings may become significant to the case.**

The following structures will describe each of the functions in the previous Matrixs.

Self Funded Vs. Fully Insured Plan

Self Funded Plan	Fully Insured Plan
Reserve Fund Potential Retention of Funds For Good Claims Experience Reserves Retained by the Plan Sponsor Not The Insurance Company	Reserves & Profit To Insurance Company
	Projected Claims
Aggregate Stoploss Premium	Pooling Charges
Specific Stoploss Premium	Administration Fees
Administration Fees	Profit Margin & Overhead
Agent / Broker Fees	Agent / Broker Commissions
Management Fees	Taxes Municipal, Surplus lines

Fixed Costs   Variable Cost   Carrier Profit

This chart shows the break down of the structure of a Self Funded Plan and a Fully Insured Plan. The Self Funded Plan provides an upside for retention of dollars as well as reduces the fixed cost known as hard dollars. In the fully Insured Plan there is no upside as you have twelve (12) cancelled checks, one for each month of the plan year, to show for the health plan which is **all** fixed cost or hard dollars and the insurance company owns the plan.

This chart is designed to give the examiner an understanding of the difference in a self funded plan and a fully insured plan as an overview. As an examiner providing the investigative approach, should have an excellent understanding of this difference based on the knowledge, education, training, and experience required for forensic investigation of the various types of Medical Plan Structures.

Information Request

At this starting point the examiner should request a copy of the Plan Documentation. This document will provide information on the Plan and the Parameters of the Plan. This request if determined to be a type of self funded plan, (Spaggregate, Self funded with Stoploss Protection or Fully Self Funded), should include a request for the Administrative Service Agreement or Administrative Service Only Agreement. Each of the requested documents will be discussed later during the examination of information.

A check list of information needed is provided to guide the examiner through the process by utilizing the vendor disclosure and Forensic Decision Mapping. The information request can be expanded based on the vendor relationships.

Anatomy of a Medical Plan

Anatomy is often looked at from a medical perspective for analysis or dissection of the human body to find out the disease, malfunction, examination for cause of conditions or death in the utilizating analytical tools and procedures. The examiner has the education, training and expertise from formal education in the field. Another coorrelation would be an automobile mechanic which analyzes vehicles based on their education, training and experience. The mechanics utilize various analytic tools as well as manuals for the anatomy of the various vehicles. The forensic examiner in the anatomy of a medical plan has the education, experience, training and analytic tools and procedures for this dissection. The basis for each area of expertise and anatomy shows that each profession has specific training and analytic tools and procedures established. The following will look at the Anatomy of a Medical Plan with coorelation to the various parts of the human anatomy since this example is relatable.

Recently, a question arose from a neurosurgeon in a conversation to explain how forensics is used in a medical plan. The explanation was quite simple, putting the plan in terms of a body.

The Pan is the body. Supporting the body are majorand minor organs as well as a support system. The major organs are the Plan Sponsor, Agent / Broker / Consultant, Contract Administrator, Stoploss, Managed Care, Network, PBM as an example. The minor organs support the major organs to allow them to function efficiently. These would include the individuals working within each of the major organs (cell structure), software used by each of the major organs (blood circulation), agreements / contracts for the supply of nutrients for each of the major and minor organs to function. Each of these major and minor organs have a circulatory system which is what continually feeds the Plan to have an optimal function. In medical terms homeostasis, the natural tendency to maintain a steady and normal internal environment.

When the internal environment for the plan gets a "bacteria or viral infection", then a diagnosis and corrective measures need to be made. Sometimes these infections are very minor and others times are major and life threatening to the plans survival. It is important for the forensic investigator to find the "bacteria or viral infection". The Body (Plan) may have suffered a significant illness or trauma from one of the major or minor organs. If the plan cannot survive, then an analysis of its "death" must be determined.

The forensic investigator must use a **methodical process** to complete a full autopsy of the body (plan). This includes the full dissection of each of the **major organs,** (Plan Sponsor, Agent / Broker / Consultant, Contract Administrator, Stoploss, Managed Care, Network, PBM), the **minor organs**, (the individuals working within each of the major organs (cell structure), software used by each of the major organs (blood circulation), agreements / contracts for the supply of nutrients for each of the major and minor organs to function), and the circulatory system.

When looking at the medical plan there are many areas which make up the operation of the plan. Each of the components are vital to the proper management and integrity of the plan. In the Forensic Investigation of a Medical Plan each of these areas are discoverable in their design, contractual arrangements, cost to the plan, compensation paid and outcomes.

The dissection of the medical plan and the findings will provide information or data on what caused the problem. These finding may be easily found and somewhat minor; however it may require significant investigation as the problem if it's major and possibly life threatening to the Plan (body). Sometimes the remedy is simple by corrective measures and the problem may not be life threatening or other findings may show a terminal problem based on multiple organ failure.

The following example shows the anatomy of a medical plan, the body, major and minor organs and the circulatory system for the medical plan. This is just an overview and is designed to be added to as the investigative medical plan forensics examines the evidence.

The anatomy of a self funded medical plan on the surface may look complicated but, breaking it down to the component level provides a means for analytics and forensics to evaluate and determine risks.

Everything in the anatomy leads to validation or invalidation by other supporting documents and data. The following is a relational base utilized by this author. In your practice you may want to use a different relational base that is able to be understood in the analytics provided in your practice.

Relational base for analytics

Plan - is the body of the self funded program
Plan Sponsor - The Brain
Plan Document - Heart
Contracted Administrator - Liver
Stoploss - Pancreas
PBM - Rt Lung
Managed Care - Lt Lung
PPO Network / Medicare + - Nose
Agent/Broker/Consultant - Ears
Accounting - Eyes
Aggregator - Spleen
PBM Auditor - Rt Kidney
Medical Claims Auditor - Lt Kidney

Each of these body parts in a self funded plan has a specific function and circulates the information to other corresponding body parts to allow the body to function in a homeostasis environment. Each of the functions provides the necessary circulatory system. All are connected to the Plan / Body. Problems occur when there is a failure of one of the organs due to a bacteria or virus. Many times the bacteria and or virus may be hard to detect and diagnose. It is the role of the Forensic Examiner to find the problems and provide remedies and or solutions to fix the problems.

There are times when the Forensic Examiner will find specific issues and provide the objective information and solutions to fix the Plan. There are also times when the Forensic Examiner will find areas so serious it jeopardizes the function of the Plan and or is so serious it can disrupt the purpose of the plan. To find the underlying problem a dissection is needed. Every part can be dissected and evaluated for solutions. Thus, solutions can be presented and sometimes a new alternative will be found.

It is important for the examiner to recognize the various problems and be able to provide solutions. Some of the more serious problems may included hard/soft fraud, theft, greed, money laundering, bank fraud, insurance fraud and embezzlement to name a few. As an examiner you will need to recognize each of these, and when found, provide the objective documentation for review by the hiring entity. No part of the plan is exempt from the examination.

As an examiner it is vital that all agreements and documentation are read completely and understood. If there is something you do not understand or defining terminology used, seek clarification in writing. This means going to the source for clarification. Remember *"you get exactly what you do not ask for!"*

By understanding the anatomy of the medical plan the investigator can dissect each of the parts and position the start of the investigation using the "Forensic Decision Mapping" to prepare the stage for a methodical analysis. There is a relational structure in the medical plan which leads to the validation or invalidation by supporting documentation and data to reach the "objective facts" in providing the basis for presentation.

Understanding the process and the investigation documentation a summary of the findings can be presented in a methodical and comprehensive report. Remember who your report is for and who the possible audience will be both currently and in the future. Keep the report and presentation of the facts simple for those who will be reviewing the findings.

Anatomy of a Medical Plan

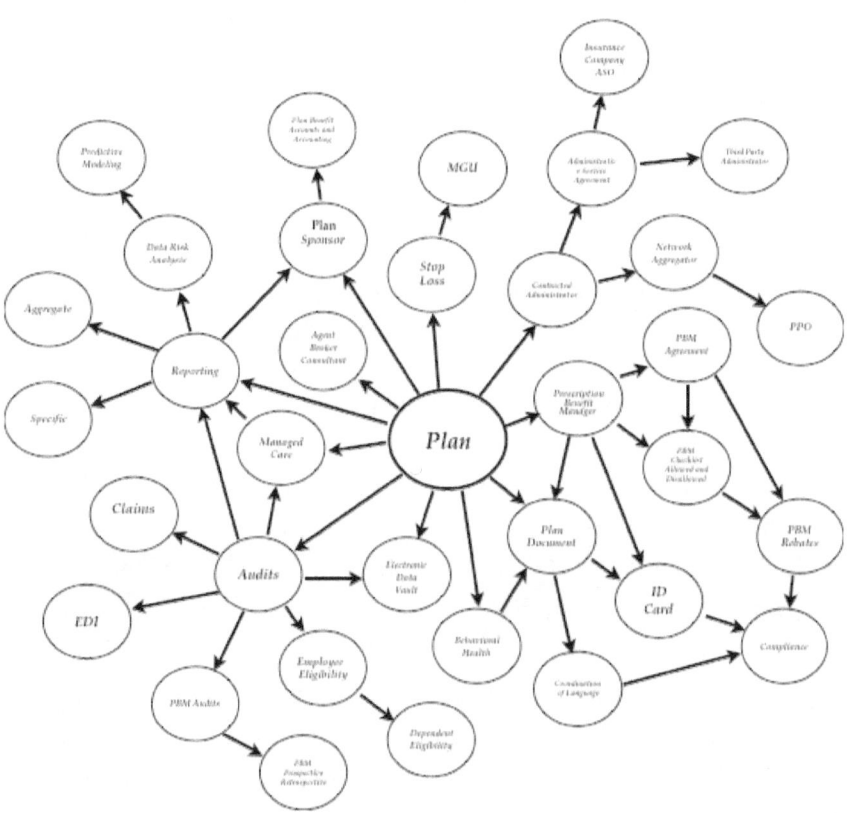

The above chart is a fundamental structure of the anatomy of a Medical Plan. As you progress in the field of Medical Plan Forensics, this structure will be expanded to reflect new integrated parts as changes occur in the medical plan environment by either market or government requirements. Thus, it is important to view this as a guide that can and will be expanded in the practice of Medical Plan Forensics.

There are new reporting requirements for medical plans due to the Affordable Care Act (ACA). These governmental requirements as added by HHS (Health and Human Services) as well as the IRS (Internal Revenue Service) as part of the Affordable Care Act are checks and balances for adherence to the ACA. These mandates are to asses those organizations who are compliant or non-compliant with the ACA. These requirements are to assess the fees, taxes and / or penalties and are designed to receive funds to support the ACA. It is important for the forensic examiner to remove the subjective opinions when validation of the facts are applied.

These governmental requirements are being evaluated in the courts by challenge of the validity in their application. The following is an example of one of the challenges to the ACA. The decision on this can have an major effect on the ACA. The following is a case in front of the Supreme Court of the United States of America.

"KING V. BURWELL (U.S. SUP. CT.)

King v. Burwell is a challenge to a key component of the Patient Protection and Affordable Care Act ("ACA"), a landmark law dedicated to achieving widespread, affordable health care. The ACA provides that individuals can purchase competitively-priced health insurance on American Health Benefit Exchanges ("Exchanges") that may be managed by either the States or the federal government. It also authorizes a federal tax credit for low- and middle-income individuals who purchase insurance on the Exchanges. The Internal Revenue Service ("IRS") issued a regulation confirming that the federal tax credit is available to all financially eligible Americans, regardless of whether they purchase insurance on a state-run or federally-facilitated Exchange.

The plaintiffs in King filed a lawsuit in the United States District Court for the Eastern District of Virginia, challenging the IRS rule on the ground that the ACA authorizes tax credits only for individuals who purchase insurance on state-established Exchanges. The ACA opponents argue, among other things, that the purpose of the tax credit provision is to induce States to set up their own Exchanges, under penalty of withdrawal of those credits and subsidies if States chose to allow the federal government to operate Exchanges in their stead.

The attorneys who represent the plaintiffs in the King case brought a similar lawsuit in the United States District Court for the District of Columbia. On January 15, 2014, the district court in that case, <u>Halbig v. Burwell</u>, ruled in favor of the IRS. The plaintiffs in Halbig appealed, and on February 14, 2014, CAC filed an amici curiae <u>brief</u> in the United States Court of Appeals for the District of Columbia Circuit supporting the federal government. That brief was filed on behalf of members of Congress who led the enactment of the ACA, including then-Senate Majority Leader Harry Reid and House Minority Leader Nancy Pelosi, as well as state legislators who served during the period when their state governments were deciding whether to create their own Exchanges.

On February 18, 2014, the district court in King, like the district court in Halbig, rejected the plaintiffs' arguments and granted the government's motion to dismiss the case. The plaintiffs in King appealed the decision to the United States Court of Appeals for the Fourth Circuit, and on March 21, 2014, CAC filed an amici curiae in the Fourth Circuit, again on behalf of members of Congress and state legislators.

On July 22, 2014 (in an opinion authored by Judge Roger Gregory and joined by Judges Stephanie Thacker and Andre Davis), the Fourth Circuit held that the IRS regulation confirming that tax credits and subsidies are available to individuals purchasing health insurance through the federal as well as state Exchanges was a "permissible exercise of the agency's discretion." Concurring in a separate opinion, Judge Davis noted that the ACA challengers' "cramped" reading of the statute was "not supported by the legislative history or by the overall structure of the Act," and concluded that "a holistic reading of the Act's text and proper attention to its structure led to only one sensible conclusion: The premium tax credits must be available to consumers who purchase health insurance coverage through their designated Exchange regardless of whether the Exchange is state or federally-operated."

The same day that the Fourth Circuit issued its ruling in King, the D.C. Circuit, by a 2-1 vote, issued a contrary ruling in Halbig. The D.C. Circuit's opinion in Halbig was subsequently vacated when the full D.C. Circuit agreed to re-hear the case en banc.)

On July 31, 2014, the plaintiffs in King filed a cert. petition asking the Supreme Court to hear the case, which the Court granted on November 7, 2014. (In light of the Court's decision to review King, the D.C. Circuit issued an order holding Halbig in abeyance pending the Court's disposition of King.)

On January 28, 2015, as in the lower courts, filed an amici curiae was filed in the Supreme Court on behalf of current and former members of Congress who were actively involved in the debates over the ACA and more than 100 current and former state legislators, all of whom were active in their states' deliberations about whether to create their own state-based Exchange. Like briefs in the Courts of Appeals, the brief here explained that the purpose of the tax credit provision iwas to facilitate access to affordable insurance through the Exchanges, not, as the ACA opponents argue, to incentivize the establishment of state Exchanges above all else, and certainly not to thwart Congress's fundamental purpose of making insurance affordable for all Americans. The brief demonstrates that there is no evidence in the legislative history of the ACA to suggest that Congress ever intended or communicated to the States that the availability of the tax credit depended upon the establishment of a State Exchange. In fact, it showed the opposite was true: everyone, including amici members of Congress, understood that tax credits would be available to purchasers on all of the Exchanges.

Further, state government officials never understood the tax credits to be limited to state-run Exchanges. Rather, as the state legislator amici know from their own experiences, the States considered many factors in deciding whether or not to set up their own Exchanges, and the possibility that not setting up a state-run Exchange would result in the loss of tax credits to the State's citizens was never one of those considerations.

The Court is scheduled to hear oral argument on March 4, 2015."

Source: www.theuscontitution.org - KING V. BURWELL (U.S. SUP. CT.)

The Forensic Examiner must keep abreast of the challenges to keep current when evaluation of medical plan requirements are tested in the courts which may or may not implicate a change in the application of the facts. These additions or changes become part of the Anatomy of a Medical Plan.

Stoploss - Risk Management

What is medical Stoploss coverage?

Medical Stoploss is an insurance product which provides protection against catastrophic or unpredictable losses. It is purchased by employers / plan sponsors who have decided to self-fund their employee benefit health plans, but do not want to assume 100% of the liability / risk for losses arising from the plans. Under a Medical Stoploss policy, the insurance company becomes liable for losses to the plan sponsor that exceed certain limits called deductibles.

Who is the insured?

A significant difference between Medical Stoploss and conventional employee benefit insurance is that Medical Stoploss insures only the employer / plan sponsor. *Medical Stoploss does not insure employees.*

It is important to understand Stoploss Insurance and its basis for risk management for the self funded plan. The Stoploss is basically broken down into three categories:

1. Specific Stoploss
2. Aggregate Stoploss
3. Attachment Point (Funding Factors)

These three basic components of a self funded plan normally constitutes 90% or more of the cost of the self funded health plan. With the attachment point / funding factors having the largest portion of the application of the costs. To put this in perspective, The "Vendor Fees and Agent, Broker and Consultant fees" are typically less than 10% of the total cost of the self funded plan when utilizing the "New Matrix". The Stoploss Premiums for specific and aggregate are normally less than 20% of the total cost. The attachment point / funding factors are normally 70% or more of the total cost of the plan.

Since Stoploss is an insurance product, a careful, methodical approach is applied since this one component is normally regulated by the Department of Insurance and has a potential for fraud to be committed against or by it. This is why it is important when analyzing the Stoploss, very strict comparisons for language between the Stoploss agreement / contract. The plan document, the administrative service agreement whether a TPA or an ASO, should be very well documented as well as the disclosure for compensation paid to any vendor to the self funded health plan. The detail of the information request by the forensic practitioner becomes very important for the proper gathering of any and all documentation including notes, emails, letters or memos to name a few for application of full disclosure.

What is the role of the plan document?

The plan document defines the benefits offered to the employees and is critical in determining the pricing of the Stoploss policy. Because the employer has great latitude in designing the plan, there may be elements in the document that are not included under the Medical Stoploss coverage. The covered portions of the plan document must be approved by the Medical Stoploss underwriter in order to effect the Stoploss coverage. Changes in the plan document after its initial approval must also be approved before their inclusion in the Stoploss coverage.

It is important to review the Stoploss Agreement to make sure it coordinates with the Plan Document. The area of importance is the basis of discounting of claims via the PPO (Preferred Provider Organization) contract and the stated discounting allowed in the Stoploss Agreement. Many times there is a difference in the two agreements. Coordination of these agreements are vital to avoid disputes in Specific or Aggregate claims as to the discounts to be utilized between the Stoploss Carrier and the Plan. This coordination will allow the proper structure in discounting when a loss is defined for eligible expenses.

How is loss defined?

Expenses are determined to be eligible for reimbursement based upon two criteria:

- The expenses must be eligible under the Benefit Plan as approved by the Stoploss Carrier.
- The loss must be covered under the covered expenses definition in the Stoploss policy.

How is the level of Stoploss Coverage Limits Determined?

The amount selected by an organization for a specific and an aggregate Stoploss requires careful consideration. The organization will be "self-insuring" the losses of the group up to these points. These amounts, along with the claims experience of the group, will also be scrutinized carefully by the underwriting department of the insurance company to determine the Stoploss coverage the carrier is willing to write.

How do I know how much to set the Specific Stoploss Deductible for the Plan?

As a rule of thumb for determining the level at which a Plan Sponsor should cap the self funded liability is to set the Specific Deductible from

5% to 15% of the total expected annual health plan claims. The size of the group can also be a factor.

Remember the specific deductible is set for each covered individual in the plan. The difference between $0 up to the Specific Deductible chosen is the funding structure used for the plan or commonly known as the Aggregate. Note: Make sure the Specific Stoploss has *Specific Advancement* and the Aggregate has *Accommodation* as provisions of the agreement.

The following is extracted from an actual Stoploss Agreements. Other agreements will be similar to these agreement provisions.

Specific Advancement

ADVANCED SPECIFIC PAYMENT BENEFIT

The Company will pay an Advanced Specific Payment Benefit to the Policyholder for any Incurred Claims payable under the terms and conditions of the Policy. The following conditions must be met for this benefit to be payable:

1. The claim must be incurred by the Policyholder for services otherwise payable under the Policy.
2. The Policyholder must make a written request for an Advanced Specific Payment Benefit.
3. The Policyholder must pay the provider(s) of service an amount equal to the Specific Deductible applicable to the Covered Person for which the claim is incurred, plus $2,000.00 for the initial claim.
4. All premiums due under the Policy must be paid currently to the end of the month for the same month the Advanced Specific Payment was requested. The Advanced Specific Payment Benefit will not be payable for any claims eligible for payment during the 31-days preceding the date of termination of the

Policy. The Advanced Specific Payment Benefit will be payable to the Policyholder in an amount equal to the remaining unpaid balance of the claim for which the Policyholder is liable, and for which benefits are payable under the Policy, subject to the Maximum Benefit for Specific Losses shown in the Schedule of Benefits.

Accommodation

"Accommodation is a fee which is paid as an option for the stoploss which reduces the exposure to the plan. Accommodation is based on the aggregate funding (soft dollars). (The aggregate is the cash within the plan to pay claims). This is based on the funding factors per category, (employee, employee children, employee spouse and family) and multiplied by the the counts / participation in each category per month for a aggregate to the plan. The accommodation allows for the plan to be exposed to only the aggregate through the current month plus previous months to which it has been exceeded. If the specific deductible is $50,000 per member then the cash on a member to meet claims prior to the specific stoploss is stoploss deductible. This amount is aggregated each month to reduce exposure to the plan as a whole. A premium is charged which is known as the Aggregate premium.

(3) ACCOMMODATION PROVISION. Accommodation shall be provided for only those claims for which reimbursement is provided under the tenns ofthe Treaty and are not in excess ofthe Specific Retention Amount. The Reinsurer shall determine for each month of coverage during the Treaty Period whether the cumulative total of Claims Paid to date by the Employer exceeds the Accumulated Aggregate Retention Amount or the accumulated pro rata portion ofthe Minimum Aggregate Retention Amount, if greater. Ifso, the Reinsurer shall pay to the Employer the difference. if more than the greater of 1.5% of the estimated Aggregate Retention Amount or $1,368,786, by which the cumulative total of Claims Paid exceeds the Accumulated Aggregate Retention Amount or the accumulated pro rata portion

afthe Minimum Aggregate Retention Amount, if greater. The total amount of Accommodation made under this Agreement shall never be more than the amount by which such Claims Paid during the Treaty Period exceeds the Accumulated Aggregate Retention Amount and shan never be more than the overall aggregate limit of $1,OOO,OOO. Accommodations shall be repaid to the Reinsurer as provided below.

(4) REPAYMENT OF ACCOMMODATION. Repayment ofthe Accommodation shall be made as follows. After an Accommodation has been paid, the Employer shall begin making monthly repayments ofthe total outstanding amount of Accommodations starting with the first month in which Claims Paid by the Employer for that month are less than (a) the Monthly Aggregate Retention Amount and the Employer's Claims Paid for that month, or (b) the total amount of Accommodations to be repaid. Monthly repayments shall continue during the Treaty Period until all outstanding Accommodations are repaid. At the end of the Treaty Period, the total amount of outstanding Accommodations is immediately due and must be repaid within 15 days of notice by the Reinsurer to the Employer of the amount to serve as fmal repayment under this Agreement. Failure of the Employer to repay any Accommodation as provided in this paragraph shall result in the assessment of a penalty of 2% per month computed on the total amount of Accommodation to be repaid.

(5) SETTLEMENT.

(a) At the end ofthe Treaty Period, the amount of any Accommodation not repaid shall be deducted from the payment of any reimbursement otherwise due the Employer under the terms ofthe Treaty. Payment of the remainder of any reimbursement due the Employer shall be made as provided in the Treaty.

(b) Operation ofthe provisions ofthis Article, for PUll'OSes of calculating the amount of Accommodation, will be determined on the basis of each Treaty Period. No Accommodation amount to be repaid to the Reinsurer shall be carried over into a subsequent Treaty Year but will be settled as provided in this Article.

(6) TREATMENT OF ACCOMMODATION. The Accommodation provided under this Agreement shall be an obligation of the Employer for which no interest shall be charged and shall be repaid as provided herein. The Accommodation is neither a loan nor an advance on any payments to be made pursuant to the Treaty. Any Accommodation shall at all times be considered funds of the Reinsurer foi which the use by the Employer of such funds is authorized by this Agreement. The Reinsurer shall have preference over all other claimants for the return of any Accommodation made under this Agreement. The Employer shall be liable for all costs and expenses, including reasonable attorney's fees, incurred in the collection of any amount of Accommodation outstanding.

(7) FEE FOR AGREEMENT. The Employer agrees to pay a fee of $2.08 per employee per month during the period this Agreement is in effect. This fee is due and payable on the first day of each Treaty Month or, if premiums are paid annually, on the first day of each Treaty Period."

Each Plan Sponsor and self funded health plan will have their tolerance level for risk. The following chart will show conservative risk limits from the low end to the high end. The plan sponsors may want to go outside of these parameters.

The following table is structured to help in setting the Specific Deductible based on group size.

Number of Covered Employees	Minimum Suggested Specific Deductible	Maximum Suggested Specific Deductible
25 - 49	$10,000	$30,000
50 - 75	$15,000	$40,000
76 - 100	$20,000	$50,000
101 - 150	$25,000	$75,000
151 - 250	$30,000	$150,000
251 - 500	$55,000	$225,000
501 - 1000	$80,000	$300,000
1001 - 3000	$125,000	$500,000
3000 +	$175,000	$500,000

Carriers have their own structures however, through my experience, the above table should be very accurate with the minimum and maximums for most carriers.

Medical Stoploss is an insurance product which provides protection against catastrophic or unpredictable losses. It is purchased by employers / plan sponsors who have decided to self-fund their employee benefit health plans, but do not want to assume 100% of the liability for losses arising from the plans. Under a Medical Stoploss policy, the insurance company becomes liable for losses that exceed certain limits called specific deductibles which has a correlation to the Aggregate Attachment Point. This is a "Risk Management Tool" for the Plan and Plan Sponsor.

Medical Stoploss is available in two-forms: specific and aggregate.

Specific Stoploss is the form of excess risk coverage that provides protection for the employer against a high claim on any one individual. This is protection against abnormal severity of a single claim rather than abnormal frequency of claims in total. Specific Stoploss is also known as Individual Stoploss. Specific Stoploss coverage provides protection for the losses relating to a "specific" claim, once it has exceeded the pre-determined level, such as $50,000, during the plan year. Claims for specific stoploss reimbursement can be submitted to the insurance company as soon as the claims exceed the Self funded level, which is sometimes referred to as the deductible.

Aggregate Stoploss provides a ceiling on the dollar amount of eligible expenses that an employer would pay, in total, during a contract period. The carrier reimburses the employer after the end of the contract period for Aggregate claims. A number of variations are available for each of these two products. Generally, all but the largest employers will want to protect their plan with both Specific and Aggregate Stoploss coverage. Occasionally, circumstances may be such that Specific Stoploss by itself will fulfill the employer's need for protection.

Aggregate Stoploss coverage provides coverage only if the combined losses for all claims exceed the attachment point selected by the Insured entity at the time aggregate coverage was purchased. This amount is usually *125* percent of the expected losses for the group. These claims are generally submitted at the close of the contract period. It is possible to negotiate a monthly Stoploss or retention with an insurance carrier, which usually apportions the annual retention over the 12-month period according to the level of claims anticipated each month.

What do the terms incurred and paid in a Stoploss contract mean?

Contracts can be done for specific periods of time. These periods are defined in the application and the eventual contract. They are expressed in the following fashion:

12/12, 15/12, 12/15, 24/12 and other variations can be done to meet the requirements of the plan. The first number is the period of time which a claim is incurred and considered eligible for payment. The second number is the period of time allowed for the claim to be processed and paid. So, a 12/12 contract based on a calendar year is defined as the claim is incurred from January 1, to December 31, and paid from January 1, to December 31, of the same plan year. If one of the numbers is in excess of 12 such as 15/12 this means the claims are incurred from October 1, to December 31, and paid from January 1, to December 31, of the same plan year.

There is a significant difference when utilizing a run in contract 15/12 for Stoploss and a run out contract 12/15 for Stoploss.

Run in allows for capturing the claims in the previous three months to be paid in the current 12 months. Run out allows for claims incurred in the current 12 months and paid in the following 3 months.

By using a "run-in" contract a gap exists for claims which are considered specific claims for the previous plan year but will not be applied to the previous Stoploss contract due to not being received in the current contract period,(considered IBNR - incurred but not received), thus, the potential exists for those claims not being reimbursed by Stoploss due to the incurred date and received in the current plan year.

The example:

12/12 Contract

A claim is in excess of the current Stoploss contract but not received in the current Stoploss contract. Example: Current specific Stoploss deductible is $25,000 - claims have been incurred in the current plan year exceeding the Stoploss deductible by $10,000. Additional claims were incurred in the current contract period but not received and applied to the new contract period. The $10,000 will not be applied to the current contract period and is not applied to the new contact period. This $10,000 is then the responsibility of the plan as it is not applied to the Stoploss or aggregate in the current contract or the new contract period. The cost to plan is $10,000.

15/12 Contract

A claim is in excess of the current Stoploss contract but not received in the current Stoploss contract. Example: Current specific Stoploss deductible is $25,000 - claims have been incurred in the current plan year exceeding the Stoploss deductible by $10,000. Additional claims were incurred in the current contract period but not received and applied to the new contract period. The $10,000 will not be applied to the current contract period but is applied to the new contact period. This $10,000 is then applied to the Stoploss and aggregate in the new contract period. Potential cost to plan is $10,000 as it is now used to meet the specific deductible in the new contract period.

12/15 Contract

A claim is in excess of the current Stoploss contract but not received in the current Stoploss contract. Example: Current specific Stoploss deductible is $25,000 - claims have been incurred in the current plan year exceeding the Stoploss deductible by $10,000. Additional claims were incurred in the current contract period but not received and applied to the new contract period. The $10,000 will be applied to the current contract period, but is excluded from the new contact period. This $10,000 is then applied to the Stoploss and aggregate in the current contract period. Potential savings to plan is $10,000 as this is reimbursed by the Stoploss company.

Terminal Liability Option (TLO)

It is important to understand the provisions of the Stoploss contract for both the specific and aggregate coverage. Some 12/12 contracts will offer a Terminal Liability Provision (TLO). Understanding the TLO is important as it can only be utilized when the self funded plan is terminated and the plan sponsor ceases to offer a self funded plan. The following example is designed to define some common language for a TLO.

The plan will pay any reimbursements presented by the terms of the policy, for expenses covered under the plan that are incurred during the policy term and paid under the plan during a 90 day period beginning at the end of the policy term if all of the following conditions have been met.

1. The Terminal Liability Option has been in force continuously during the entire plan period; and
2. It ceases to offer a self insured plan at the end of the policy term; and
3. The Plan Sponsor gives notice of such termination at least 30 days before the end of the Stoploss policy.

When reimbursements become payable under the terms of this Option, the Aggregate Attachment Point will be recalculated retroactive to the beginning of the Policy Term, using the Aggregate Factors shown in the Terminal Liability Option.

Specific stop rates will continue for two months beyond the termination of the policy.

The differences in the applicable Stoploss Contracts has an impact on the renewals going forward.

A 12/15 Stoploss contract provides a better basis for renewal. The current contract is independent and allows for better competition with regard to underwriting. The claims incurred in the previous contract period stops with the current contract period and allows for better competition for Stoploss for the new contract period since the underwriter is only concerned with the claims incurred at the basis of the new Stoploss contract.

A 15/12 contract is normally utilized when the initial contract is a 12/12 contract. The Stoploss must now estimate the amount of run in allowed and may limit the amount of claims by dollar amount to be eligible for the run in contract. Any new renewal is based on estimates by the underwriter of the exposure they are willing to take for the run in contract.

Each of the Stoploss contract provisions has their place in the overall scheme of the self funded plan. The Plan Sponsor must know the risks involved and make a decision as to the risk exposure they are willing to take. It is important for the Agent / Broker / Consultant to explain the various risks for the Stoploss contract provisions in allowing the Plan Sponsor to make the best choice for their plan.

What does an Admitted and Non-Admitted Insurer / Carrier mean?

Admitted Insurer - Insurer licensed to do business in the state which the insured exposure is located.

Non-Admitted Insurer - Insurer not licensed to do business in the state in which the insured exposure is located.

Submission of Request for Quote to the Stoploss Carrier.

The preparation of the information to submit to the Stoploss carrier will determine how well rates will be calculated. Utilizing the proper format with the pertinent information for this request can mean a significant difference in the rates and factors quoted by the Stoploss Carrier. The preparation of this request gives the "story" of an employee benefit plan. This must be factual information for each category required by the Stoploss Carrier for quote evaluation.

As stated above: *The detail of the information request by the forensic practitioner becomes very important for the proper gathering of any and all documentation including notes, emails, letters or memos to name a few for application of full disclosure.* This information is a basis for validation of information sent to the "Underwriters" in providing a Stoploss quote. Additionally, the source of the information should be contacted as well. The source may be an insurance company, a TPA, the Plan Sponsor. The comparison of this information can uncover a potential for fraud based on the secondary transmission of the original information provided to the Agent, Broker or Consultant. Included in this is the "Census" information which utilizes a Date of Birth (DOB). Validation of this information is very important since it is one of the easiest to manipulate to show a younger average age for the group which the underwriters will use in determining the cost of risk for the Stoploss insurance and the Attachment point / funding factors. *Note: when a deviation of this information is found it should be noted as it is normally an* **intentional act** *versus a clerical error when the original submitted census from the employer states one thing and the Agent, Broker or Consultant retransmission of the data states something different.*

It is important to view all information used for the accuracy of transmission to the underwiters for their risk assessment in determining the Stoploss rates and factors. Utilizing false or misleading information and transmission of this information for Stoploss insurance purposes in determining risk assesment for rate determiniation is considered **"insurance fraud"**.

Checking the Status of the Stoploss Carrier.

It is important to check with your States' Department of Insurance to validate the approval of the Carrier as an Admitted Insurer. Simply go to the Department of Insurance web portal for specific State or Commonwealth to check the status of the Stoploss Carrier. In addition, it is important to check the AM Best Rating of the carrier. Simply go to the AM Best web portal and loginfor free and register.

Stoploss Agreement / Contract Provisions

Many Stoploss agreements / contracts have limitations which are important to understand as they may limit the reimbursements /

accommodations of the amounts exceeding the specific deductible or aggregate. These provisions may be amended by mutual agreement to structure a seamless basis between the Plan Document, Administrative Service Agreement and Stoploss Agreement.

When dealing with health plans, you should be aware of potential pitfalls in coverage which exist with the plan documents, Stoploss policies that insure them and the PPO Agreements. Falling into one of these pitfalls can be messy and painful. When a pitfall occurs, it is likely that lawsuits and a bad experience of the self insured plans will occur.

The main issue for self funded plans are the agreements between plans and the various entities serving the Plan, and the lack of coordination of the agreements. The lack of coordination between the plans, Stoploss carriers, third-party administrators, PPO networks and hospitals can cause litigation over the agreements.

Stoploss Agreements Don't Coordinate Language with Self funded Plans

The agreements between a Stoploss carrier and self funded plans must be coordinated. The agreement with the Stoploss Carrier should be carefully read to understand how they determine eligible claims and the reductions from the gross claim submitted is calculated for an allowed claim. This understanding can help avoid litigation.

Many times a TPA will tell clients the Stoploss carrier will mimic the Plan Document and all claims are reimbursed that exceed the Stoploss Limits are eligible. This is simply not a true statement in todays environment.

It is important to keep all correspondence received from any consultant, broker or agent if they are making statements that the claims in the plan are totally covered by the Stoploss Agreement. Keeping this correspondence may not help when the claim is denied but will help in filing an E & O Claim against the consultant, broker, agent or TPA for recovery of the difference in the claim allowed and the amount denied by the Stoploss Carrier.

When a Stoploss insurer denies a request for reimbursement under the Plan, the first reaction is to accuse the Stoploss Carrier for not upholding the agreement. For example, the plan administrator may state they paid the claims based on the plan document. The TPA will point to the Stoploss Carrier for the failure to reimburse the plan based on the Plan Document. This problem between the Plan Document and the Stoploss Agreement is due to the non coordination of the Plan Document Parameters and the Stoploss Agreement Parameters that creates a deficit in coverage for eligible claim reimbursement to the Plan. Simply stated these two agreements do not match up.

It is important to review the exclusions in the Plan Document and the Stoploss Agreement. Many of the exclusions are not coordinated. Thus, problems can and will occur. Some exclusions in the Stoploss Agreement states illegal acts are excluded. The Plan Document may state that felonious acts are excluded. These two are very different and the Plan may pay because the act was not felonious but the Stoploss carrier will exclude the claim because it is an illegal act. A good example in this instance is an individual covered by the plan is driving and is prosecuted under a DUI due to the individual being involved in an accident which is a result of the DUI. A DUI is normally considered a misdemeanor which is not a felony but is considered an illegal act. The TPA will apply the Plan Document Provisions and pay the claim since this was not a felony in this example. The Stoploss Carrier will deny the claim due to their language of an illegal act. This is a deficit in the coordination of the Plan Document and the Stoploss Agreement.

Defining a Claim Payment

Another area which can be problematic for the Plan and the Agreement with the Stoploss Carrier is how a claim payment is defined.

This can be viewed from the differences of what the TPA understands as a paid claim and what the Stoploss Carrier defines as a paid claim. The importance is understanding the Stoploss Agreement as to the definition of the Paid Claim. By the TPA not recognizing or understanding the agreement with the Stoploss Carrier on a Paid Claim can give rise to a denied Stoploss Claim and litigation which will involve the Plan Sponsor, the TPA and the Stoploss Carrier. The Stoploss Carrier will hold to the Agreement executed by the Plan Sponsor for the eligibility of the claim. The TPA is the entity which will have a responsibility of the claim. The Administrative Service Agreement with the TPA and the Plan Sponsor now comes into play. The Plan Sponsor will most likely litigate against the TPA for recovery of the denied claim from the Stoploss Carrier.

Payments can be defined in many ways. One understanding of the Payment is the date the TPA processed the check. Another is the date the check is mailed. And lastly is the date the check was received. Stoploss Carriers will validate which ever the case may be for their reimbursement of a Stoploss Claim based on their agreement. Thus, depending on the Language in the Stoploss Agreement the claim may not be covered by the Stoploss based on their definition of a Paid Claim. Thus, the coordination of the Plan Document, Stoploss Agreement and TPA Check Processing are vital.

Many TPA's will use a fulfillment company for the checks to be issued and mailed. Depending on the definition used by the Stoploss Carrier a problem can occur when the TPA has issued the checks to be printed and the fulfillment company processes the approval by the TPA for the checks to be printed and mailed two days later. Why is this example important? The Plan Year may end on December 31 and the checks submitted to the fulfillment company are on December 28 but do not get processed and mailed until January 2. The Stoploss Agreement may state the checks must be issued and mailed by December 31 to be considered for reimbursement. Thus, claims would not be eligible under the Stoploss Agreement.

The PPO now enters into the Deficit problem

The coordination of the Stoploss Agreement, Plan Document and the Preferred Provider Organization (PPO) agreement is a major concern for the basis of allowable discounting on a claim. Most TPA's will pay the claims for In-Network or PAR claims based on the Plan Document and the agreement with the PPO. However, the Stoploss Agreement may only allow the claim to be paid on the basis of Usual, Customary and Reasonable (UCR) price. The difference can cause the potential loss of Stoploss protection on a contract with the carrier.

The importance of the coordination of these agreements is vital to the allowance of claims recognized by the Stoploss Carrier, the contract with the PPO on the agreement with the Plan Sponsor, Plan Document and the TPA. The TPA may process the Participating (PAR) claims based on the Plan Document and the discounts received from the PPO based on the contract. However, the Stoploss Carrier may only recognize the UCR table to be applied to the claim for reduction. So the question arises, "What is the difference?"

The PPO contract may apply a discount of say 20% to the claim. In this example we will look at a claim of $1,000 for simplicity.

Description	Claim Using PPO	Claim Using UCR
Gross Claim	$1,000.00	$1,000.00
PPO Discount Applied	20%	
UCR Table Applied Allowable		$500.00
Eligible Claim	$800.00	$500.00

The above example the Stoploss Carrier would recognize on the $500 Eligible Claim. The TPA may submit the $800 Eligible Claim. The difference is $300 in the eligible claim.

Also this example the Plan Sponsor based on the language of the Stoploss Agreement would lose the additional $300 as an allowable reimbursement, even though the claim was paid based on the PPO Agreement. This difference in the discounting can allow the Provider under the PPO Agreement to balance bill the Participant for the difference. This will also have an effect on the Plan as it may be considered a Breach of Contract with the PPO Agreement and may give rise to litigation and termination of the PPO Agreement. Just imagine if this claim was $100,000 or $1,000,000 instead of $1,000. The effect could be catastrophic.

The Stoploss Carrier is justified based on their contract and the Plan Document. Remember the Stoploss Agreement normally allows for the Carrier to have an independent audit of the claims and identify the UCR Table Rates that should be applied to the claim. This is independent of the TPA who may be performing audits of the claims.

Coordination of these agreements can avoid potential problems for all concerned.

PPO Agreement Contract and Terms

The terms of the plan document may state a plan must be prudent with the assets of the plan, and each claim should be carefully processed before any payment is made to a Provider. However, the PPO agreement may not be stated the same way.

The agreements under a PPO state that you do not have a right to audit the claims. Their agreement is based on a fixed discount amount to be paid on a timely basis which is normally 30 days. Remember, the client to the PPO is the Provider which is given the right to audit the claim. This is known as a self audit.

A problem arises with the PPO Agreement vs the Plan Document language. The agreement will state the claim must be paid in accordance with the PPO Agreement. If the Plan does not pay in accordance with the agreement then the PPO can pursue litigation for Breach of Contract. The PPO will normally win in this situation. Thus, the plan will pay based on the PPO Agreement, the Stoploss agreement will reimburse on the UCR and the Plan and or Participant will have the balance to pay. This creates a deficit in the coordination of the claims.

The Stoploss Agreements draft their agreements to allow the lowest cost for the reduction of the claim. This is taking the PPO Discount or the UCR Table Amount and allowing reimbursement on whichever calculates to be the lowest cost for allowance of reimbursement under the Stoploss Agreement.

Therefore, the agreements must be read in their entirety. The proper consulting and drafting of the agreements to coordinate all parties to an agreeable language can prevent litigation and problems for all concerned.

Thus, choosing the right Stoploss carrier is more than just a rate. Selecting the lowest rate which is done by many TPA's, Consultants, Brokers and Agents can lead to problems. The best way to avoid these problems is to have a qualified person review the agreements which have the fewest deficits in their application. Many times language can be drafted as an addendum to these agreements for simplification and coordination to make sure all parties are reading from the same page.

Investigation of Stoploss Reimbursements

The investigation requires the Forensic Analyst to gather all the information available to develop an objective based opinion. This opinion must be "FACT" based. Information will also be needed from the Contracted Administrator on the reimbursement(s) being evaluated. The information from both must be applied first independently and then viewed utilizing comparative analytics for gaps, errors and omissions by and between the two sets of objective data. Additionally, as mentioned above, the Stoploss agreement must be reviewed for any limitations imposed. The best method to use for this investigation is the Forensic Decision Mapping for Stoploss Reimbursement as this will provide the methodical approach to the data received to process for the objective based opinion. This Forensic Decision Mapping also allows the analyst to show the flow of work for the data analytics to the hiring entity as well as provideing the basis for writing the report. If the forensic analyst is being hired as a testiying expert, then the decision mapping using simple terms to describe the findings will work in laying out the information to a jury as they will understand the picture and flow of objective data used to develope the objective opinion.

The use of a second Forensic Decision Mapping for Accounting is normally utilized to show the objective facts for the health benefit account. This is important to use for validation of the flow of money, validation of deposits, payments and various transactions. This data is also used to compare to the information received from the Contracted Administrator and Stoploss Carrier with regard to the financial validation of transactions as they apply to the investigation at hand.

The following is a claim based on an out of network provider for surgery on a participant, the Contracted Administrator provision on a percentage of savings, the aggregator who provided the negotiation for the percentage of savings and the resulting denial of a portion of the percentage of savings.

Claim Example for Stoploss Partial Denial

Example 1

Plan Sponsor - Stop Loss Carrier (Participant Specific Stop Loss Reimbursement worksheet)

Description	Amt 1st Submission 2/29/16	Amt 2nd Submission 5/4/16	Difference 5/4/16 vs 2/29/16
Coinsurance	$57,838.33	$58,201.13	-$362.80
Co-Pay	$35.00	$104.40	-$69.40
PPO Discount	$122,984.76	$123,628.16	-$643.40
Other (Aggregator Fee)	$8,642.94	$8,642.94	$0.00
Total	$189,501.03	$190,576.63	-$1,075.60

In submission #2 on 5/4/16 the amount submitted for Stoploss Specific Reimbursement $2,261.70. The Amount reimbursed on 5/9/16 check 1560 is $1,186.10. The difference is $1075.60 as Discounts and Adjustments. There was not any detailed information for the Discounts and Adjustments per the reports or a copy of the submission to analyze the differences.

Example 2

The following is a work up of a claim billed by a Hospital to the self funded plan. The hospital does not participate in Networks.

Claim	Total Claim	
The Hospital	$279,534.72	
Aggregator Negotiated Reduction	$172,859.03	Claim Reduction
Adjustments	$7,999.09	Ded., Co-Ins, Co-Pays
Total Reduction Allowed	$180,858.12	
Allowed Claim	$98,676.60	
Less Stop Loss Ded	$25,000.00	Plan Paid
Total for Stop Loss Reimb	$73,676.60	
Stop Loss Reimbursement	$65,033.69	Stop Loss Paid
Not Allowed - exceeds 25% Savings	$8,642.91	
Not Allowed by Stop Loss	$8,642.91	Plan Paid

The information for this filing is from January 1, 2016 through February 29, 2016. To figure the savings to use as a base for the Aggregator Billing, the check registers were reviewed for the above dates on Aggregator payments (Jane Doe Claim). The total amount in the check register for the Aggregator is $51,857.71. To get the basis of the dollars for the savings: $51,857.71 / 30% = $172,859.03. The chart listed below will summarize the difference. Stoploss allows 25% of savings for application to Stoploss reimbursement. The Contracted Administrator added per the Administrative Service Agreement the extra 5% to the fee for savings calculation. This amount was above the allowed threshold of the Stoploss Contract and is a fee paid directly to the Contracted Administrator for the processing of this particular sequence of claims on the hospital for the Plan on the Participant. Thus, the payment to the Contracted Administrator is a fee and is not part of the claim. Due to the agreement between the Contracted Administrator and the Aggregator, the Aggregator bills the 30% as the fee for services for reduction of the claim. The Aggregator then pays per agreement the Contracted Administrator the 5% as compensation.

The chart below summarizes the information from Example 1 and 2 above.

Percentage	Savings	Billed	Allowed by Stop Loss	Difference Not Allowed
30%	$172,859.03	$51,857.71		
25%	$172,859.03		$43,214.76	
5%	$172,859.03			$8,642.95

Through the Aggregator the health plan saved a net of:

$172,859.03 - $51,857.71 = **$121,001.32 (Extremely good savings for the Plan)**

Observation / Recommendation

The Plan Sponsor should either contract directly with the Aggregator for services or renegotiate the terms of the Administrative Service Agreement. The Contracted Administrator provides their services for an administrative fee of $20 per employee per month. This fee is by contract and is to encompass the processing and adjudication of all the claims. The above is a claim on the differences not allowed of $8,642.95 is compensation to the Contracted Administrator and is excluded from the specific Stoploss and aggregate Stoploss as it is considered exgratia as an excess fee. All of the negotiation and preparation and defense of the claims listed above are handled by the Aggregator not the Contracted Administrator. The Contracted Administrator received the negotiated claim from the Aggregator and processed it as a normal claim but received a significant fee for processing these claims from The Hospital. The Contracted Administrator added the clause for percentage of savings:

Bill Audit-Claim Negotiations-Wrap PPO Network Fees-30% of savings;

The Forensic Analyst needed to view **all of the information**, and the data was received and applied to the various forensic decision mappings for analytics. This included gathering all of the infomation from the Plan Spnsor, Contracted Administrator and the Stoploss Carrier. Information includes all detailed information, accounting, claims, billings and payments as they apply to the incident at hand.

The above is a summary report The actual full report would include the Forensic Decision Mapping and exhibits, plus work for processing and objective opinion.

Pharmacy Benefit Management (PBM)

The PBM is an important component to your Health Benefit Plan. Selection of the proper PBM can significantly impact the dollars spent for prescriptions. The PBM will have a network of participating pharmacies for the participants to utilize for their prescription needs.

In reviewing the PBM, due diligence must be done. The PBM agreements are one of the toughest agreements to analyze due to the complexity of their wording. By understanding the wording of the agreement the plan sponsor can make a good decision on the choice of the PBM to be utilized for their health benefit plan. Not understanding the wording of the agreement can have a significant increase on the cost of prescriptions to the plan.

In the author's experience prescription cost to a plan can range from 12% to 78%. This is a significant spread impacting the claim cost to the health benefit plan.

When plan sponsors have been asked the question: Is your PBM processing the pharmacy claims according to the terms of your contract? The most common answer is I think so, but I'm not sure. The reason for this is many plan sponsors and contracted administrators have just accepted that the billing from the PBM is accurate without mistakes. This is due to the simple math with complicated rules which produce processing errors. Many contracted administrators accept what the

PBM bills as accurate. However, when the proper analysis is done on a prospective basis in analyzing the prescription benefits against the check list, errors will be found. The is no official oversight of the PBM activities. By implementing a compliance analysis both on a prospective basis and a retrospective basis for the plan check list as well as the PBM agreement to the plan as a strategy, dollars will be found as errors which should be paid back to the plan as restitution of overcharges and non compliant charges according to the agreements with the PBM.

Note: The prescription benefit cost to a plan has a range of 10% to as much as 80% of the claim costs to the plan. Thus, it is important to manage this area of the health benefit plan.

The prospective audit of PBM claims for compliance against the checklist and PBM agreement is one of the best methods to control the errors in the billing of the prescriptions. To achieve this compliance on costs an audit of the claims should be done prior to the payment of the gross invoice sent by the PBM for payment. This audit procedure is based on every claim on a line by line basis comparing the claim to the check list as well as the PBM agreement. There are very important issues with this auditing of the PBM claim. The PBM must agree to provide the various tables to the auditing firm used for the prescriptions in the billing cycle to determine the cost basis used for the claims. A comparison and analysis is done to insure the claims are processed accurately for the tables utilized. In addition, the claims are processed against the agreement between the plan and the PBM for compliance of dispensing time tables as well as quantities of the prescriptions dispensed. These are just two of the components used in the analysis. If a PBM refuses to provide the appropriate information for this procedure then one should look for a PBM that is agreeable and make PBM changes.

When the prospective auditing procedure is utilized, then the audited net bill is paid to the PBM for the claims with the audit results. The PBM then has the right to review those claims which were reduced by the audit and appeal to the plan under the appeal process in the time frame with in the health plan document based on its language. This appeal must have the reasoning and show on an objective basis why the gross claim billed is accurate. There are some PBM's that will state you must pay the gross claim, present your audited claim results to them for their determination of the differences in the claims. This procedure is not in the best interest of the plan sponsor as your dollars may never be refunded to your plan. The PBM will also have many delay tactics which are implemented such as changing the individuals in their PBM who are reviewing the audit which starts the time frame over and over as they will change individuals internally on this process.

In the prospective audits I have reviewed they always, 100% of the time, find errors.

This prospective audit procedure implemented as part of the operations of the plan on prescription claims will reduce the loss ratios, retain dollars to the plan and produce a better structure. By sharing this procedure with the Stoploss carrier the results will help in the underwriting of the plan and in the reduction of the specific and aggregate Stoploss insurance as well as the funding factors.

Note: There are many companies providing "PBM Auditing" in the market. When choosing the company to use in the prospective auditing, the audit must be on a line by line basis and not just a sampling. The line by line audit is a valid audit and is an effective structure used with the PBM. The PBM will not acknowledge a sampling audit as there is no real validation. The choice of the auditing company chosen must be independent and not affiliated with any PBM. In the retrospective audits reviewed have found errors 100% of the time.

The prospective auditing does have a cost for this service to the plan. However, my experience shows, the return on investment (ROI) is significant in the application of this service.

Many companies will choose to do a retrospective audit. The retrospective audit can be performed for up to seven years on past claims. This audit must have the same structure as the prospective audit. The difference is the gross claims have been paid to the PBM and the plan is requesting the restitution of the over charges. Remember, the PBM has already received the funds and will not want to make restitution. There will be delay tactics and the PBM will want to negotiate a reduced amount for the restitution. Remember, this is health benefit plan dollars to be returned to the Plan and not the PBMs money. The amount of dollars found in the line by line audit can be significant.

The auditing of the claims for contract analysis will reveal the following areas but is not limited to these errors and exclusions found.

Processing Errors that may be found -

Brand vs Generic Assignment
Comparison to Usual and Customary
Zero Balance
Day Supply Limits - Retail and Mail Order
DAW - Dispense as Written
AWP - Average Wholesale Price % Variance

Cost Errors that will be found -

MAC - Maximum Allowable Cost list compliance
True AWP (Average Wholesale Price) cost
AWP (Average Wholesale Price) % Discount
Dispensing Fee

Exclusion Errors that will be found -

NDC - National Drug Code Analysis
Drug Category
Claim Date Range
Member ID and Status

In addition to the audits, there are other dollars which may be found in the analysis and forensics of the PBM structure and agreements with the TPA and/or ASO Insurance agreements as contracted administrators to the plan. There are many revenue streams associated with the agreements. Some of the revenue sharing agreements between the contracted administrator and the PBM are listed in the chart below.

The following are some areas for revenue sharing between the PBM, Contracted Administrator and / or the consultant, broker or agent. These areas of revenue sharing may be disclosed or non-disclosed compensation.

Category	Description
Administrative Fees	Fees may be added to the this as compensation.
Per Script Fees	Fees may be added to the this as compensation.
Rebates	Sharing of the rebates which are basically refunds to the plan.
Card Fees	Normally with the contracted administrator as renumeration for producing the ID Cards.
AWP Spread	A % may be shared as compensation.
Dispensing Fee Spread	A % may be shared as compensation.
Generic or Mac Spread	A % may be shared as compensation.

Some of these fees will be difficult to find, however, with the Forensic analytics applied, these can be found and disclosed to the Fiduciaries of the health benefit plan.

As a Plan Sponsor / Fiduciary in selecting the PBM which will work as a true partner to the plan, there are procedures to put in place for this selection.

The first is to recognize the current information with regard to the Plan and the claims processed are the property of the plan. Thus, having the proper request for this information and being provided in the proper format are essential for the analytics to be completed. This information is processed and analyzed utilizing the proper tools and distributed to the current PBM community for response to an RFP by providing the parameters for the proposals to be received and processed for the purpose of making the proper selection. The selection made will have the PBM agree to the contract terms set forth by the Plan Sponsor / Fiduciary in the application of the PBM provision to the health benefit plan. Then as the Plan Sponsor / Fiduciary the agreement is between the Plan and the PBM. Full transparency of the PBM is put in place and the prospective auditing procedures are agreed upon by contractual agreement as a checks and balance to this provision of the health benefit plan.

Parties / Vendors to the Plan

The following are the basic vendors to the plan. It is important to complete this information form for investigative work to begin. This list can be expanded to encompass all of the vendors to the plan. This information will be used to structure the Forensic Decision Mapping and compile disclosed and non disclosed compensation. This list provides the entities who need to be contacted to request initial information and additional information as the investigation continues.

Plan Sponsor

This is the organization who has sponsored the plan. This is also the fiduciary of the plan.

Plan Sponsor:	Plan Sponsor Name
Contact:	
Address:	
City, State Zip:	
Phone:	
Email:	
EIN:	

It is always a good idea to search with the Secretary of State for verification of the Plan Sponsor as a legally registered entity in the State. It is also advisable to print the current annual filing submitted by the plan sponsor. It is better to have too much information than to be without the information in providing a complete forensic investigative report.

This information will also allow the Forensic Investigator to go to the free website: http://freeerisa.benefitspro.com for the 5500 Form for the plan year(s) in question. The 5500 Form information will be utilized in the investigation in conjunction with the Forensic Dissection of Form 5500 tool.

TPA / ASO Vendor

The TPA / ASO is the contracted administrator to the plan. It is important to get the full legal name of the contracted administrator. In the preliminary information, it is important to perform a search with the Department of Insurance in the State where the plan sponsor is domiciled to validate the Administrator is licensed in the State / Commonwealth to provide the administrative services. When searching, the investigator will want to print the information and make it part of evidence.

Contracted Administrator:	TPA / ASO Name
Contact:	
Address:	
City, State Zip:	
Phone:	
Email:	
EIN:	
DOID Number:	
NPN Number:	
Licenses Held:	
Appointed by Carrier:	

Understand that not all may be required to be registered in the State to do business and provide administrative services. However, the Department of Insurance for the Domiciled state of the Plan Sponsor will require the Contracted Administrator to hold a resident or non-resident license with them. In addition, if the Contracted Administrator is soliciting or providing Stoploss as part of their service, they should be licensed as an agent / agency with the appropriate resident or non-resident license. When searching the license information it is also important to validate the Appointment by the Stoploss Carrier for the Contracted Administrator. Most states require the appointment in order to solicit the Stoploss Insurance Carrier.

Stoploss Vendor

The Stoploss carrier is providing the risk protection for the plan. It is important to research the carrier with the Department of Insurance in the state of domicile to validate the carrier is approved and admitted or non approved and not admitted.

Stoploss Carrier:	Stoploss Carrier Name
Contact:	
Address:	
City, State Zip:	
Phone:	
Email:	
EIN:	
NAIC Number:	
Approved In State:	
Policy Number:	

MGU Vendor

Many times the Stoploss Carrier will use an Managing General Underwriter (MGU) that is appointed by the carrier to underwrite the risk and provide the cost of this protection for the Plan

Managing General Underwriter:	MGU Name
Contact:	
Address:	
City, State Zip:	
Phone:	
Email:	
EIN:	

Insurance Agency / Agent Vendor

The agent is normally considered the solicitor for forensic investigation. It is important to get the full legal name of the Insurance Agency. In the preliminary information, it is important to search with the Department of Insurance in the state where the plan sponsor is domiciled to validate the Insurance Agency is licensed in the state / commonwealth to provide the sale of insurance products. In addition, if the agent is part of the agency, the agent should be listed as Designated to Act on behalf of the Business Entity. The investigator will want to print the information and make it part of evidence.

At times there will be more than one agency and agent involved in the case. Be sure to get the information on each of these entities. The form below shows the information needed on each. If there are more, simply expand the form to include the addition entities.

Agency Firm 1	Insurance Agency Name
Contact:	
Address:	
City, State Zip:	
Phone:	
Email:	
EIN:	
DOID:	
NPN:	
Licenses:	
Appointed by Stoploss Carrier:	

Agent Agency 1	Agent Name
Contact:	
Address:	
City, State Zip:	
Phone:	
Email:	
EIN:	
NPN:	
Licenses:	
Appointed by Stoploss Carrier:	

Consulting Firm / Consultant Vendor

It is important to get the full legal name of the Consulting Firm and or Consultant. Many consultants are not attached to a firm. In the preliminary information, it is important to search with the Department of Insurance in the state where the plan sponsor is domiciled to validate the Consultant is licensed in the state / commonwealth as a Consultant and Agent if they provide the sale of insurance products. Not all states have a requirement for an individual to be licensed as a consultant due to no consultant licenses issued by the state or commonwealth. However, many states do have this requirement and an individual can not call themselves a consultant unless properly licensed.

In addition, if the consultant is part of the consulting firm, the consultant should be listed as Designated to Act on behalf of the Business Entity. When searching, the investigator will want to print the information and make it part of evidence.

Consultant Firm	Consulting Firm Name
Contact:	
Address:	
City, State Zip:	
Phone:	
Email:	
EIN:	
DOID:	
NPN:	
Licenses:	
Appointed by Stoploss Carrier:	

Plan Consultant	Consultant Name
Contact:	
Address:	
City, State Zip:	
Phone:	
Email:	
EIN:	
DOID:	
NPN:	

Licenses:	
Appointed by Stoploss Carrier:	

Managed Care Vendor

This firm provides the Utilization Review / PreCertification / Disease Management / Case Management and many other areas as a vendor to the plan.

Managed Care Firm:	Managed Care Firm
Contact:	
Address:	
City, State Zip:	
Phone:	
Email:	
EIN:	
Credentialed Certifications:	

Aggregator Vendor

This firm provides multiple services for the plan. They provide Electronic Data Interface (EDI) functions for claims, repricing of claims for PAR Claims (In Network) and Non-PAR Claims (Out-of-Network). In addition they will provide claim scrubbing, bill review and other service to the plan for efficiencies. Many times the PPO Vendor will contract with the Aggregator and the Aggregator will provide the PPO to the Plan. It is important to get the PPO Vendor information being utilized by the plan. In some instances there may be more than one PPO Vendor to the Plan due to the geographic distribution of the

Plan Sponsor's participants. Expand the PPO Network information as needed until all networks utilized are recorded.

Aggregator Firm:	Aggregator Firm Name
Contact:	
Address:	
City, State Zip:	
Phone:	
Email:	
EIN:	

PPO Vendor

PPO Network 1:	PPO Network Name
Contact:	
Address:	
City, State Zip:	
Phone:	
Email:	
EIN:	

PBM Vendor

This vendor provides the network for the Prescription Access to the plan. This vendor is very important as the claims from this vendor may be as much as 30%+- of the claims to the Plan.

PBM:	PBM Name
Contact:	
Address:	
City, State Zip:	

Phone:	
Email:	
EIN:	

PBM Auditing Vendor

This vendor provides auditing services to the plan. This is normally done on a prospective basis. Not all plans use a PBM Auditing Firm.

PBM Auditing Firm	PBM Auditing Firm Name
Contact:	
Address:	
City, State Zip:	
Phone:	
Email:	
EIN:	

Add additional vendors to the plan until all have been captured. This information will be valuable in starting the process on the investigative forensics process.

Example

The following is an example of a search on the Agent / Broker / Consultant and the Stoploss Carrier. For simplicity purposes, I will use myself as this will have each of the licenses described for the Agent / Broker / Consultant.

Plan Consultant	Consultant Name
Contact:	F. Randall Childers, Jr., CFC, DABFE
Address:	227 Rolling Ridge Way

City, State Zip:	Simpsonville, KY 40067
Phone:	(502) 643-8739
Email:	Randall_childers@me.com
EIN:	SSN: xxx-xx-xxxx
DOID:	390690
NPN:	7209157
Licenses:	Life, Health, Consultant Life and Health, Administrator
Appointed by Stoploss Carrier:	Yes

From this information it is known this individual's resident state / commonwealth is Kentucky. We will do a search on the Kentucky Department of Insurance website http://insurance.ky.gov/Agent/Default.aspx to get the balance of the information. Follow the prompts for the search.

This search does not contain the Insurance Agency or Consulting Firm as this individual is independent. However, if the Insurance Agency or Consulting Firm does come up then search on the Insurance Agency and/or Consulting Firm as done with the Agent / Broker / Consultant and complete the information. As an investigator, if there is additional information you find necessary, then add it to your form and complete the information.

Search Results Agent / Broker / Consultant

Department of Insurance 1/13/13 6:32 AM

Kentucky.gov — KY Agencies | KY Services | Search [Kentucky.gov] for Search Terms [Search] [Go]

Kentucky Department of Insurance

eServices Secure Website

↗ denotes external link

Search Home   Agent Licensing

Agent/Agency Search Details as of 1/13/2013

Name : Childers Jr, Frank Randall
DOIID : 390690
NAIC NPN : 7209157

[View Affiliations] [Continuing Education Information]

License - Line of Authority Information

Status	Residency	Class	Line of Authority	Active Date	Inactive Date	Appointments	License Expiration Date	Home State
Active	Resident	Administrator	Not Applicable	3/13/1992			3/31/2015	
Active	Resident	Agent	Health	6/28/1984			3/31/2015	
Active	Resident	Agent	Life	6/28/1984			3/31/2015	
Inactive	Resident	Agent	Prepaid Dental Plan	4/7/1998	3/1/2001			
Inactive	Resident	Agent	Health Maintenance Organization	11/10/1997	3/1/2001			
Active	Resident	Life & Health Consultant	Not Applicable	5/13/2008			3/31/2015	

*If a status is Pending, Pending Replacement, or the record displays Affidavit on File, click on them for more details.

License Renewal Information

Class	Invoice Date	Response Due / Expiration Date	Response Received Date	Payment Received Date	Renewal Complete
Administrator	01/15/2013	03/31/2013	10/13/2012	10/13/2012	Yes
Agent	01/15/2013	03/31/2013	10/13/2012	10/13/2012	Yes
Life & Health Consultant	01/15/2013	03/31/2013	10/13/2012	10/13/2012	Yes

NOTE: Licensee may renew up to 6 months prior to Next Compliance Date. Licensees subject to CE must complete CE requirements before Next Compliance Date in order to successfully complete the License Renewal Process.

Address Information

Type	Address
Residence	Not Public Information
Business / Home Office	227 Rolling Ridge Way Simpsonville, KY 40067

No Internet Information on File

Privacy Policy | Disclaimer | Accessibility Statement   Font Size [10] [12] [14]

Copyright © 2010 Commonwealth of Kentucky
All rights reserved.

file:///Users/randallchilders/Documents/Book%20Employer%20Choice%20...0Plan%20Forensics/Department%20of%20Insurance%20Childers.webarchive   Page 1 of 1

From the information contained in this search result, the following can be obtained. This individual has resident licenses of Agent Health, Agent Life, Administrator and Consultant Life & Health. The completed form will look like the following:

Plan Consultant	Consultant Name
Contact:	F. Randall Childers, Jr., CFC, DABFE
Address:	227 Rolling Ridge Way
City, State Zip:	Simpsonville, KY 40067
Phone:	(502) 643-8739
Email:	Randall_childers@me.com
EIN:	SSN: xxx-xx-xxxx
DOID:	390690
NPN:	7209157
Licenses:	Agent Health, Agent Life, Consultant Life & Health, Administrator.
Appointed by Stoploss Carrier:	Fidelity Security Life Insurance Company.

Lets assume the Stoploss carrier is Fidelity Security Life Insurance Company. While on the Department of Insurance website, view the Appointments with the following insurers. The results shown are:

Active	**Fidelity Security Life Insurance Company**	300466	Agent - Health	2/8/2011	
Active	**Fidelity Security Life Insurance Company**	300466	Agent - Life	2/8/2011	

The result is this individual is appointed with the Stoploss Carrier.

When searching for the agent / broker / consultant in a State other than the resident state based on where the Plan Sponsor is domiciled, as an investigator, go to the Department of Insurance website and perform a search. This will confirm or deny the agent / broker / consultant as properly licensed to do business in that state or commonwealth for soliciting / selling the insurance product. As an investigator, the form will be expanded with additional columns to show the results of the search.

Always print the search results as this will normally have a date stamp as in the example above in the top right hand corner 01/13/13 6:32 AM. This will also provide a reference point in the investigation should a second search show different information.

Search on the Stoploss Carrier. The order of the searches does not matter the order of the search to get the results as they will be the same.

Stoploss Carrier:	Fidelity Security Life Insurance Company
Contact:	Richard F. Jones
Address:	3130 Broadway Blvd.
City, State Zip:	Kansas City, MO 64111-2452
Phone:	(816) 756-1060
Email:	
EIN:	43-0949844
DOIID:	300466
NAIC Number:	71870
Approved In State:	Kentucky
Policy Number:	

The following is the search results from the Kentucky Department of Insurance WebSite and the information above has been filled in. This is public knowledge.

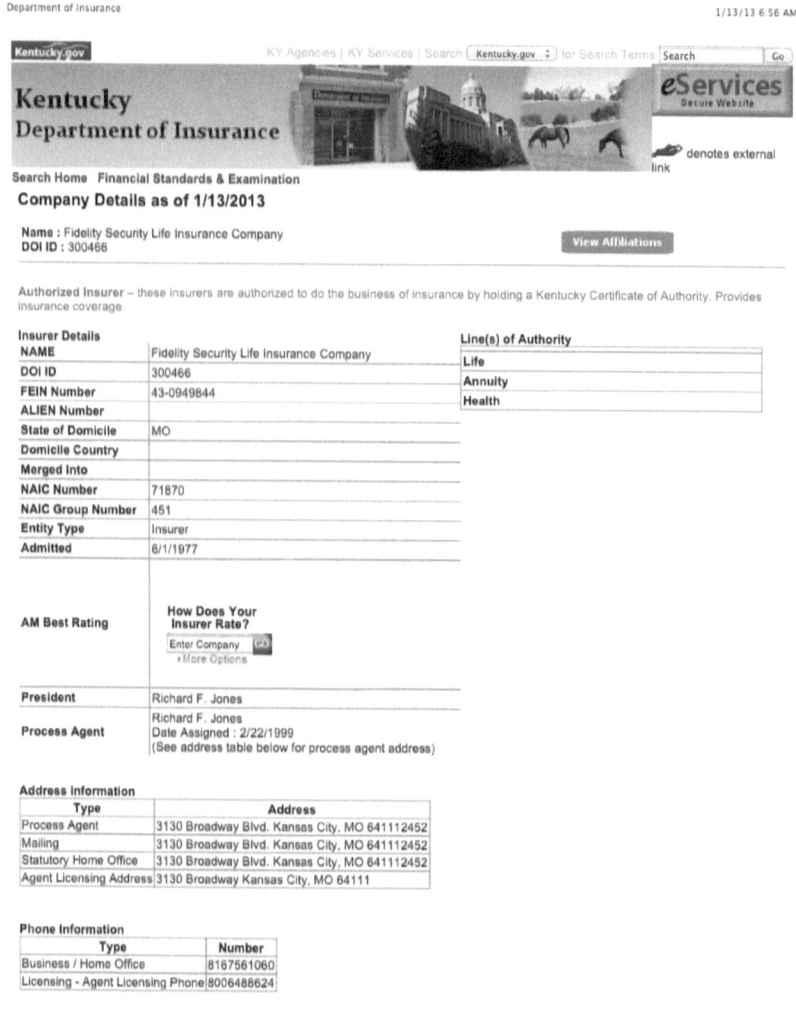

Search Results Fidelity Security Life Insurance Company

Additionally, note there is an AM Best Rating portal built into the WebSite. Use this to obtain information and print the results. The following is the result on the Stoploss Carrier.

Result AM Best Search

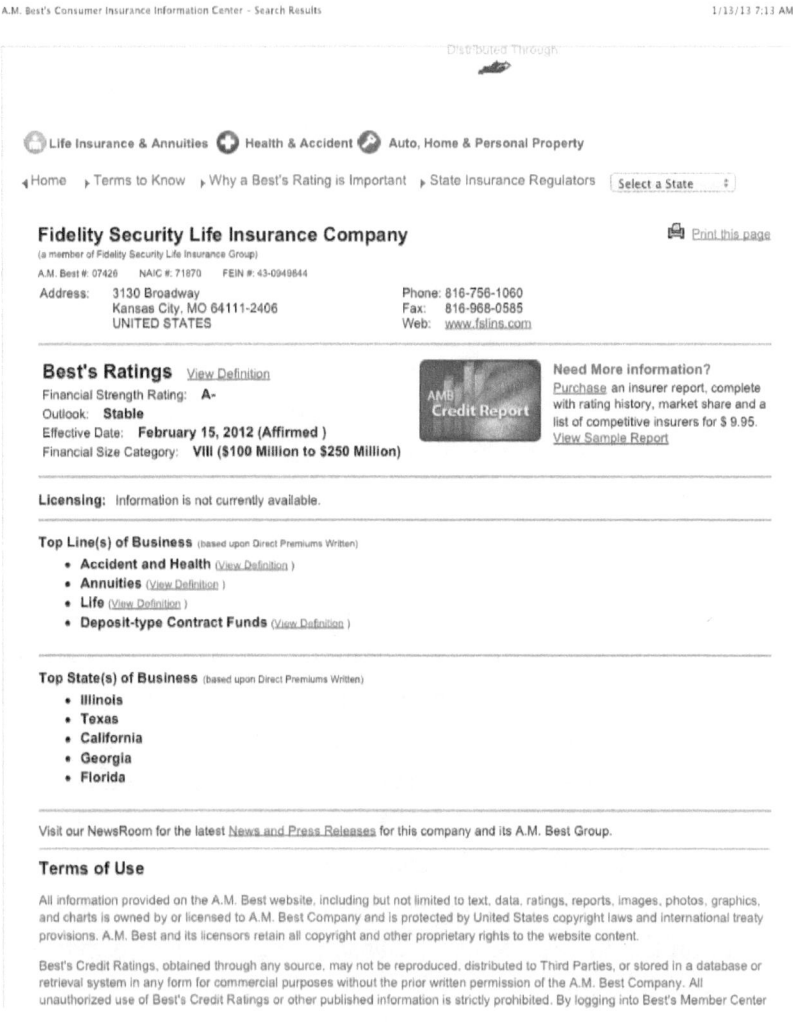

Always print the search results as this will normally have a date stamp as in the example above in the top right hand corner 01/13/13 6:56 AM, DOI and 01/13/13 7:13 AM, AM Best Report. This will also provide a reference point in the investigation should a second search show different information.

At the bottom of each search result page is the full website address for the search. Note this as there are many searches done in a forensic investigation for reference points.

This should provide the information needed to do searches with the Department of Insurance WebSites. One note, not all websites are as easily used as the Kentucky Department of Insurance. Some of the websites are very cumbersome to use, but take the time to get the information needed. Call the DOI if the information is not readily available.

As each of your searches are completed and the information compiled, I normally will start a binder with tabbing on the Vendors to the Plan. Be sure you allow for expansion due to additional vendors being found, providing services to the plan that may become vital information to the investigation.

One of the additional searches done on the Agent / Broker / Consultant is the Continuing Education. The issue in the case may be on a particular area. This search will allow the investigator to see the most recent Continuing Education on the Agent / Broker / Consultant. This may become vital to the investigation based on the training and education received in a specific area of practice. If you find you will need more information with regard to the continuing education, simply call the Department of Insurance and request the information. The state of residence on the Agent / Broker / Consultant is where the Continuing Education will be found.

Note: Based on the case, you may want to request any complaints, DOI lawsuites and various other issues to help in the investigation of the entity.

Search Result Continuing Education

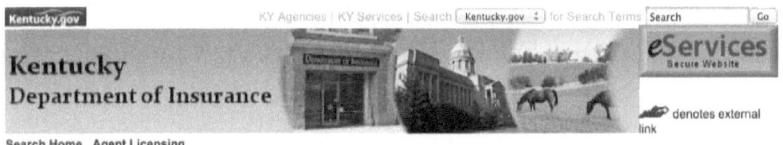

Department of Insurance   1/13/13 7:39 AM

Kentucky Department of Insurance

Search Home Agent Licensing

Agent Licensing - Continuing Education Information as of 1/13/2013

Name : Childers Jr, Frank Randall   **DOI ID** : 390690
NAIC NPN : 7209157

If a course you have completed is not listed below, please contact your CE Provider to validate that it has been sent to the Kentucky Department of Insurance (DOI). All CE Courses received by DOI are posted on the web site within (3) working days.

UPDATE FOR KENTUCKY RESIDENT LICENSEES:

- **Effective July 2005**, the Legislation required that if you are subject to Continuing Education you must complete three (3) hours of Ethics in order to be compliant for a biennium, which is defined as the last day of your birth month and even or odd year based on your birth year.
- **Effective July 1, 2006**, your Continuing Education biennium compliance date will be the same as your License Renewal compliance date.
  - Continuing education requirements must be satisfied as a condition for license renewal, and will be due the same month/year that your License Renewal is due.
- **EFFECTIVE February 6, 2009**, for Licensees with a Continuing Education compliance date beginning February 2009:
  - The Twelve (12) hour **CLASSROOM REQUIREMENT has been removed;** therefore, you may now meet your twenty-four (24) hours of continuing education without the classroom restrictions.

Twenty-four (24) hours of approved continuing education must be completed during each continuing education biennium. At least six (6) hours must be directly related to any line of authority for which the agent is licensed. At least three (3) hours must be ethics each biennium.

Agent CE Compliance Date:
3/31/2013

CE Compliance Date	Ethics Hours	Ethics Complete	LOA Hours	LOA Complete	Class Carryover	Class Hours this Biennium	Class Complete	Corr. Carryover	Corr Hours	Total Carryover hours	Total CE Hours	Compliant This Period
3/31/2015	0	No	0	No	3	0	N/A	0	0	3	3	No
3/31/2013	6	Yes	16	Yes	3	14	N/A	2	8	5	27	Yes
3/31/2011	3	Yes	19	Yes	5	10	N/A	0	14	5	29	Yes
3/31/2009	3	Yes	23	Yes	3	14	N/A	0	12	3	29	Yes
6/30/2006	4	Yes	20	Yes	3	24	Yes	0	0	3	27	Yes
6/30/2004	4	Yes	20	Yes	3	24	Yes	0	0	3	27	Yes

REMEMBER:

- You must renew complete renewal application by License Expiration Date **AND** complete CE requirements on or before CE Compliance Date in order to successfully complete the License Renewal Process.
- Three (3) hours of Ethics and six 6) hours in one or more of your Lines of Authority must be completed each biennium.
- Only twelve (12) excess credit hours earned during a biennium may be carried forward as general hours to your next continuing education biennium.
- Newly licensed individuals are subject to CE and License renewal when the license ha been active for 12 months; CE and Renewal due date is defined as the last day of your birth month and even or odd year based on your birth year.

http://insurance.ky.gov/Agent/ALce.aspx?Type=1&LookupVal=390690   Page 1 of 2

Always print the search results as this will normally have a date stamp as in the example above in the top right hand corner 01/13/13 7:39 AM, Continuing Education Report.

This report, if Fraud is considered shows the individual completed the Continuing Education on: Insurance Fraud - C06381, Course Concentration: Life, Health, Property & Casualty, Kentucky Provider Name: WebCe, Inc., Date of Completion: 11/13/2011, Method of Instruction: Correspondence, Credit Hours: 6, Compliance Date: 03/11/2011.

This information confirms this is an extensive course due to the (6) hours of Continuing Education (CE) Credits. If needed for the investigation, contact the Department of Insurance and get a copy of the course approval, and contact the CE Provider, in this case WebCE and request a copy of the information and course. Due to the nature of the case, a request of the questions in the exam may be appropriate.

The information you request should relate to the issue at hand. Of course, investigations can lead to other areas of concern which on the surface may not seem important but may become vital to the case. Always follow the objective evidence, make no assumptions. Experience, Education, Training and Expertise should provide the knowledge in evaluating and following the objective data / information and provide evidence of the forensic examiners search.

This information and all information is considered discoverable meaning the information will be found with the investigation.

From this information, certain setups can be done in preparation of analytical analysis be accomplished. This information is used to set up the chart of accounts in the accounting system for the compilation of data in cost and compensation paid by the plan. The following is an example for the chart of accounts - **Expense Account**.

Expense Accounts
Bank Service Charges
Insurance Expense
Stoploss Premium Specific Premium

Stoploss Premium Aggregate Premium
Aggregate Accommodation Fee
Medical Claims
Prescription Claims
Professional Fees
Consultant Fees
Agent / Broker Fees
Medical Administration Fees
PBM Fees
PPO Fees
UR/PreCert/CM/DM/NL (This category is used for Managed Care Company fees)

The chart of accounts is **expandable** based on the data received. Each line in the chart of accounts should have a setup of the various organizations with the detailed information as documented above including the entity name, their EIN and or SSN with the contact person, address, and phone numbers and attached to the corresponding categories.

This will also provide information of the proper filing of IRS 1096 and 1099M as well as information for the reporting on the 5500 Form. These areas will be addressed later and the significance of this information.

Information Request

The information that follows is derived from specific reports requested from the various vendors. These reports are detailed to the information requested and the format to be provided in a spreadsheet format, normally, .xls and or PDF. Reports may be required from the Plan Sponsor / Fiduciary as well.

Note: you get exactly what you do not ask for!

The execution of a Business Associate Agreement (BAA) is essential with the Plan Sponsor/ Fiduciary/ Trustees of the Plan. This form should be completed and signed on the engagement of the Forensic Examiner. This will eliminate the hesitance of providing information and using HIPPA and PHI as excuses to not provide the information. This form will be included in the requests to each vendor.

In addition, it is time for inclusion of the Corporate Attorney and CPA. If the CPA firm has a forensic accountant, then this individual should be included as well. A briefing of information to this point will be given and the process to use next. The Attorney will draft a letter to each Vendor for the request of information to be provided. Information received by the Forensic Examiner should be shared with the Forensic Accountant as to the objective information of data and analysis of the data.

The following is a listing of the information which may be needed. Remember to request the information for the issue at hand. Additional information is requested as the investigation moves forward and where the objective findings may lead.

In each section a sample letter of request is included.

Note in the letters below, the items needed were the items requested. A second letter can be sent with any additional request.

Plan Sponsor

Reports to Request

1. Copies of quotes and documentation including any correspondence from Contracted Administrator and or Agent / Broker / Consultant.
2. Copies of all Plan Documents and agreements signed.
3. Copies of all billings received from Contracted Administrator and any vendor to the plan.
4. Copies of all check registers received from the Contracted Administrator.
5. Copies of all government filings such as Form 5500 with Schedules A and C. Any and all filings with regard to the medical plan for ACA compliance.

Banking Information for Plan

1. Provide copies of Plan Bank account information and all statements.
2. Provide copies of all reconciliation reports on Plan Accounts.
3. If banking for Plan is handled with a software program, download a file in .xls format of all detailed transactions entered in system and/or export for Accountant Copy.

Contracted Administrator

Reports to Request - All reports to be provided in an .xls and/or PDF.

1. Software System used in processing the claims.
2. Plan Document(s).
3. Administrative Service Agreement.
4. Agreements with all vendors to the Plan.
5. Provide **all** compensation received from each vendor to the plan where applicable. Compensation includes all fees and commissions. Please provide copies of statements and checks or check stubs for each.
6. Detailed Census Report
7. Detailed Billing Report by Month.
8. Detailed Claims Report for all claims processed by the Plan both Medical and Rx.
9. Detailed Provider Report for all providers who have been paid by the Plan.
10. Detailed Vendor Report for all vendors who have been paid by the Plan.
11. Detailed Check Register for Providers Paid by the Plan.
12. Detailed Check Register for Vendors Paid By the Plan.
13. Detailed Deposit Register for Plan.
14. Bank Statements for each month of the Plan.
15. Provide copies of any and all subrogation checks received with detail of claim(s).
16. Provide copies of all refunds from providers to the plan with detail on original claim and refund detail from provider.
17. Provide detail on all COBRA transactions with billings and checks received from participants and associated payments to the plan account.
18. Provide copies of all checks received from providers as refunds or over payments on claims. This should have claim detail with claim numbers and individual names.

19. Provide copies of submissions to Stoploss carriers with detail as well as copies of any spreadsheets used in the analysis of Stoploss carriers.
20. Provide detailed copy of 50% Specific Report.
21. Provide detailed copies of Specific claims made to Stoploss Carrier for Reimbursement and checks received from carrier.
22. Provide copy of aggregate report for plan.
23. Provide detailed copies of Aggregate claims made to Stoploss Carrier for Reimbursement and checks received from carrier.
24. Provide copies of any audits done on claims and billings for this service to plan.
25. Any potential lawsuits?

Banking Information Request

Detailed Deposit Account with Banking Information, Address, Phone, Banking Representative and Routing and Account Number. Also, include banking set up form with MICR layout and signature cards for account. Please provide account ownership information.

Detailed Checking Account with Banking Information, Address, Phone, Banking Representative and Routing and Account Number. Also, include banking set up form with MICR layout and signature cards for account. Please provide account ownership information.

If utilizing a sweep account in conjunction with the Deposit Account then provide Account with Banking Information, Address, Phone, Banking Representative and Routing and Account Number. Also, include banking set up form with MICR layout and signature cards for account. Please provide account ownership information. Provide floor used for sweep and max allowed for sweep. Include any statements on this account for earnings.

Provide all statements for accounts associated with the Plan Sponsor / Fiduciary / Trustee for XYZ Plan. If reconciliation reports are available then provide the reports for each account. If using an accounting/banking system then export to an .xls file the reconciliation detailed reports in coordination with each statement and account.

License and E&O Requests

1. Provide a Copy of the TPA or Administrator License for Resident License.
2. Provide a Copy of the TPA or Administrator License for the State of Corporate Residence for the Plan Sponsor.
3. Provide a Copy of the Life and Health Insurance License both Resident and Non Resident the State of Corporate Residence for the Plan Sponsor.
4. Provide Proof of Administrator approval from MGU and/or Stoploss Carrier.
5. Provide Proof of Appointment by Stoploss Carrier for both the resident license and non-resident license the State of Corporate Residence for the Plan Sponsor.
6. Provide a Copy of the Corporate E&O policy, crime policy and/or Bonding as an Administrator.

Note in the letter below, the items needed were the items requested. A second letter can be sent with any additional request.

Sample Letter Contracted Administrator

Administration Company **Monday, January 14, 2013**
Mr. Joe Smith, President
1234 Any Street
Any Town, State 12345

Re: XYZ Company 2009 Plan Year.

Mr. Smith,

This is a request for information on the XYZ Company for the 2009 plan year. Please provide the following information. A letter of authorization is attached from XYZ Company. Information requested is to be provided by **January 18, 2013**.

Documents

1. Software System used in processing the claims.
2. Plan Document(s).
3. Administrative Service Agreement.
4. Agreements with all vendors to the Plan.

Reports

1. Detailed Census Report
2. Detailed Billing Report by Month.
3. Detailed Claims Report for all claims processed by the Plan both Medical and Rx.
4. Detailed Provider Report for all providers who have been paid by the Plan.
5. Detailed Vendor Report for all vendors who have been paid by the Plan.
6. Detailed Check Register for Providers Paid by the Plan.
7. Detailed Check Register for Vendors Paid By the Plan.

8. Detailed Deposit Register for Plan.
   9. Bank Statements for each month of the Plan.

Thank you in advance for the information.

Sincerely,

F. Randall Childers, Jr., CFC
Cc: XYZ Company

Agent, Broker or Consultant

Reports to Request

Provide **all** compensation received from each vendor to the plan where applicable. Compensation includes all fees and commissions. Provide copies of statements and checks or check stubs for each.

License, E&O Requests, Analysis and Presentations

   1. Provide a Copy of the Agent / Broker / Consultant License for Resident License.
   2. Provide a Copy of the Agent / Broker / Consultant License for the State of Corporate Residence for the Plan Sponsor.
   3. Provide a Copy of the Life and Health Insurance License both Resident and Non Resident the State of Corporate Residence for the Plan Sponsor.
   4. Provide Proof of Appointment by Stoploss Carrier for both the resident license and non resident license the State of Corporate Residence for the Plan Sponsor.
   5. Provide a Copy of the E&O policy, crime policy and or Bonding as an Agent, Broker or Consultant.
   6. Provide copies of submissions to Stoploss carriers with detail as well as copies of any spreadsheets used in the request for quotes.

7. Provide copies of all quotes received and the analysis (spread sheets) of Stoploss carriers for this plan.
8. Provide a copy of the proposal and presentation for the medical plan.

Provide a written detail of services provided to the Plan and Plan Sponsor.

Note in the letter below, the items needed were reworded for the items requested. A second letter can be sent with any additional request.

Sample Letter to Insurance Agent

Insurance Agent   **Monday, January 14, 2013**
Mr. Joe Smith, Agent
1234 Any Street
Any Town, State 12345

Re: XYZ Company 2009 Plan Year.

Mr. Smith,

This is a request for information on the XYZ Company for the 2009 plan year. Please provide the following information. A letter of authorization is attached from XYZ Company. Information requested is to be provided by **January 18, 2013**.

1. Provide a Copy of the proper license with the Line of Authority for this case. Consultant License, Life and Health Insurance License for both your Resident state and Non Resident the State of Corporate Residence for the Plan Sponsor.
2. Provide Proof of Appointment by Stoploss Carrier for both the resident license and non resident license for the State of Corporate Residence of the Plan Sponsor.
3. Provide a Copy of the E&O policy, crime policy and or Bonding as an Agent, Broker or Consultant.
4. Provide copies of submissions to Stoploss carriers with detail as well as copies of any spreadsheets used in the request for quotes.
5. Provide copies of all quotes received and the analysis (spreadsheets) of Stoploss carriers for this plan.
6. Provide a copy of the proposal and presentation for the medical plan.
7. Provide a statement of all compensation received on the plan fees and or commissions by any party to the plan.

8. Provide a written detail of services provided to the Plan and Plan Sponsor.

Thank you in advance for the information.

Sincerely,

F. Randall Childers, Jr., CFC
Cc: XYZ Company

Prescription Benefit Manager (PBM)

Reports Requested

1. Copy of PBM Agreement and script checklist.
2. Detail report of all transactions and billing for the Plan by billing period. (Provide in .pdf and .xls format).
3. Provide report when payments on Prescription billings were received
4. Provide detailed report on *all* compensation paid. Compensation includes all fees and commissions. Please provide copies of statements and check copies for each.
5. Provide detailed reports for all Rebates received and Rebates Paid. Detailed report on rebates paid to Plan, Contracted Administrator and/or Agent / Broker / Consultant.

Note in the letter below, the items needed were the items requested. A second letter can be sent with any additional request.

Sample Letter PBM Company

PBM Company   **Monday, January 14, 2013**
Mr. John Smith, PhR
1234 Any Street
Any Town, State 12345

Re: XYZ Company 2009 Plan Year.

Mr. Smith,

This is a request for information on the PBM Billings for XYZ Company for the 2009 plan year. Please provide the following information. A letter of authorization is attached from XYZ Company. Information requested is to be provided by **January 18, 2013**.

Reports Requested

1. Copy of PBM Agreement and script checklist.
2. Detail report of all transactions and billing for the Plan by billing period. (Provide in .pdf and .xls format).
3. Provide detailed reports for all Rebates Paid to XYZ Company for the 2009 Plan Year. Provide the Date of the Check, Check Number, Amount of Check and the rebate period (example 1st qtr 2009, 2nd qtr 2009, 3rd qtr 2009 and 4th qtr 2009.

Thank you in advance for the information.

Sincerely,

F. Randall Childers, Jr., CFC
Cc: XYZ Company

PBM Auditing Company

Reports Requested

1. Copy of Auditing Agreement
2. Copy of PBM Agreement and script checklist used.
3. Detail report of all audited transactions and results per PBM for the Plan by billing period. (Provide in .pdf and .xls format).
4. Copies of all audit billings submitted for the Plan and Payments Received.
5. Provide detailed report on *all* compensation paid to the Contracted Administrator / Agent / Broker / Consultant. Compensation includes all fees and commissions. Please provide copies of statements and check copies for each.

Note in the letter below, the items needed were the items requested. A second letter can be sent with any additional request.

Sample Letter PBM Auditing Company

PBM Auditing Company **Monday, January 14, 2013**
Mr. John Doe, President
1234 Any Street
Any Town, State 12345

Re: XYZ Company 2009 Plan Year.

Mr. Doe,

This is a request for information on the PBM Auditing for XYZ Company for the 2009 plan year. Please provide the following information. A letter of authorization is attached from XYZ Company. Information requested is to be provided by **January 18, 2013**.

Reports Requested

1. Copy of Auditing Agreement
2. Copy of PBM Agreement and script checklist used.
3. Detail report of all audited transactions and results per PBM Billing (PBM Company) for the Plan by billing period 2009 Plan Year. (Provide in .pdf and .xls format).
4. Copies of all audit fee billings submitted for the Plan and Payments Received.

Thank you in advance for the information.

Sincerely,

A. Randall Childers, Jr., CFC, DABFE

Cc: XYZ Company

MGU / Stoploss Carrier

Reports requested

1. Provide copy of quote. This should include the quote with commissions and the quote net of commissions. Include with the quote with commissions the amount of taxes for surplus lines and municipal taxes and any other taxes calculated in quote with and without commissions. Use the % of taxes as well as the $ amount of the taxes for each census level. In addition provide the $ amount of commission to be paid and to whom amount is paid to.
2. Provide a copy of the submission for quote with all correspondence and detail received from the Contracted Administrator / Agent / Broker / Consultant. Provide any spread sheets submitted for census or any other documentation used in providing the quote.
3. Provide copy of signed Stoploss Agreement.
4. Provide copy of census transmitted by Contracted Administrator or Agent / Broker / Consultant used in quoting Stoploss.
5. Provide signed copy of Disclosure Statement used in quoting plan.
6. Provide copy of approval letter for Contracted Administrator.
7. Provide a statement and validation of approved carrier in state of plan sponsor.
8. Provide a copy of the appointment for each entity which includes Contracted Administrator and Agent / Broker /Consultant for approval to sell, solicit and/or receive commission/fees from Carrier.
9. Provide detailed report on *all* compensation paid. Compensation includes all fees and commissions. Please provide copies of statements and check copies for each, Contracted Administrator and Agent / Broker / Consultant.
10. Provide statement of any contingency bonuses paid to Contracted Administrator and or Agent / Broker / Consultant.

11. Provide statement of any Stoploss commission/fee paid to Contracted Administrator and or Agent / Broker / Consultant which is not calculated in the plan. This will include compensation paid on net quote.
12. Provide copies of all checks paid on the Plan for Specific and Aggregate reimbursements with detailed statement of calculation for each check issued.
13. Provide copies of any audits performed for specific claims and or aggregate claims.

Aggregator

Reports Requested

1. Provide copy of agreement with Contracted Administrator.
2. Provide report on Out-of-Network (OON) claims processed with discounts applied.
3. Provide report on OON claims negotiated with discounts applied.
4. Provide copies of billings to Contracted Administrator for payments on OON Claims repriced or negotiated with detail.
5. Provide copies of any and all compensation paid to Contracted Administrator on OON or negotiated claims with detail including each check.
6. If providing PPO PAR network repricing, provide a statement of contracted per employee per month (PEPM) charged to plan for each network with detail of billing including census used for each PPO.
7. Provide a statement of all services provided to Contracted Administrator.

Managed Care

Reports Requested

1. Provide copy of agreement with Plan Sponsor and/or Contracted Administrator.
2. Provide copy of worksheet used for services to be provided.
3. Provide statement of net PEPM fees charged for services.
4. Provide detail report on charges to plan for case management.
5. Provide copies of any and all compensation paid to Contracted Administrator or Agent / Broker / Consultant with detail including each check.

PPO

Reports Requested

1. PPO PAR network repricing, provide a statement of net PEPM charged to plan for network with detail of billing including census used for PPO.
2. Provide copies of any and all compensation paid to Contract Administrator or Agent / Broker / Consultant with detail including each check.

Sample letters provided as a guide. As the practitioner, the development of the letters for each vendor and the information to be requested is specific to each unique circumstance.

Dissection Fees

Forensic Disscetion Fees, Premiums and Compensation

The following information / disclosure forms are intended to provide an overview of the costs associated with the plan. This information is gathered from the documentation requested and received by the various vendors to the plan.

As the forensic examiner, the initial information received should be listed in the following forms based on entity. When entering the information, questions may arise for clarification. These questions should be noted under each entities disclosure as a future reference in requesting additional information and or findings. This information should be updated as objective data presents itself. Additionally, the information gathered in this disclosure is utilized in setting up the initial analysis tool to get a visual of the data presented for analytics and structure for the accounting in the chart of accounts.

The initial information may not disclose all of the parameters for compensation, cost and agreements. Thus, as the objective information presents itself a notation should be made for proper analytics and the forensic reports.

Always remember the notes you make, data received and the analytics are discoverable for the parties involved if the information is to be used. This includes but is not limited to interrogatories, discovery, depositions and court.

If you have been hired to evaluate, analyze and provide findings to a hiring entity without a court case, the information should be prepared and available as if it were going to court. It is recommended to use the following in this situation for confidentiality when communicating to the hiring entity for each document: Privileged work product should be placed on each document. Even when you have placed this on the document, the hiring entity can use this information and disclose. This is normally a decision made by the hiring entity and legal council.

Always remember, everything is discoverable!

Administrator Compensation Disclosure

This compensation disclosure is for both the disclosed compensation and non-disclosed compensation. Each of the items listed below must be completed as requested by the Fiduciaries of XXX Plan. It is in the best interest of the XYZ Contracted Administrator (TPA) or Insurance Company (ASO) to comply with this disclosure request.

Contracted Administration Fees:

The contracted administration fees for the XXX Plan is as follows: Please complete the appropriate structure with the $ PEPM or the proper % percentage. Pull this information from the Administrative Service Agreement.

PEPM	Composite	Employee	EE + SP	EE+ 1	EE+Children	Family
Composite	$					
By Census		$	$	$	$	$

% of Claims	Composite	Employee	EE + SP	EE+ 1	EE+Children	Family
Composite	%					
By Census		%	%	%	%	%

If using a % of Claims as the administrative fee, state if the % is based on the following:

__Gross Claims   __Allowed Claims   __Paid Claims

Compensation Paid From Contracted Administrative Fees

Many times compensation is paid to the Agent, Broker or Consultant. The following request is on any compensation paid from the administration fees to any Agent, Broker or Consultant. Please complete the following chart as the compensation paid whether disclosed in the Administrative agreement or not disclosed in the administrative agreement. *(This information is completed from the interview of the Contracted Administrator (CA)).*

PEPM	Composite	Employee	EE + SP	EE+ 1	EE+Children	Family
Composite	$					
By Census			$	$	$	$

% of Claims	Composite	Employee	EE + SP	EE+ 1	EE+Children	Family
Composite	%					
By Census		%	%	%	%	%

Please state whom fees/compensation is paid to:

Name:_____
Address:_____
City:_____ State:_____ Zip:_____
EIN or SSN:_____
Amount: $_____PEPM   %_____ of claims

Name:_____
Address:_____
City:_____ State:_____ Zip:_____
EIN or SSN:_____
Amount: $_____PEPM   %_____ of claims

Name:_____
Address:_____
City:_____ State:_____ Zip:_____
EIN or SSN:_____
Amount: $_____PEPM   %_____ of claims

It is important to note the CA may have been requested by the Agent/Broker/Consultant (ABC) to add to the administrative fees. The reason is the ABC does not want the Plan Sponsor (PS) to know all compensation paid to them. This information is not reported on form 5500 or Schedule A or C for payments received from the CA Administrative Fees. The only reporting is by the CA via 1099 to ABC. Thus, it is important to convey to the CA honestly and disclosure of this type of structure is in the best interest of them, the plan and PS.

Disclosure of UR/PreCert/CM/DM/Wellness Plan

The fees contracted by contracted administrator with the Managed Care Provider as contracted to the XXX Plan are: *(Enter the information from the Administrative Service Agreement).*

PEPM Gross	Composite	Employee	EE + SP	EE+ 1	EE+Children	Family
Composite	$					
By Census		$	$	$	$	$

Please state the net rate charged from the Managed Care Provider. *(This information is by requesting the copies of the billings and Agreement from the Managed Care Provider).*

PEPM Net	Composite	Employee	EE + SP	EE+ 1	EE+Children	Family
Composite	$					
By Census		$	$	$	$	$

If there is a difference in the PEPM Gross and the PEPM Net, was the difference retained by the contracted administrator? _____Yes _____No.

Was this compensation disclosed or is this compensation considered undisclosed to the Fiduciaries of the Plan? Please Explain:

Is there a sharing of this compensation to the Agent, Broker or Consultant as compensation?

Please state whom fees/compensation is paid to:

Name:_____
Address:_____
City:_____ State:_____ Zip:_____
EIN or SSN:_____
Amount: $_____PEPM

Name:_____
Address:_____
City:_____ State:_____ Zip:_____
EIN or SSN:_____
Amount: $_____PEPM

Name:_____
Address:_____
City:_____ State:_____ Zip:_____
EIN or SSN:_____
Amount: $_____PEPM

Request a report from the Managed Care Vendor (MCV) on all billings sent for processing to the CA and payments received by the MCV. This report along with the vendor payments reports and claim reports from the CA are used to validate all information is accurate by comparing payments in the reports.

For the Case Management or Large Case Management disclose the appropriate charge base:

Per Hour Rate: $_____
PEPM: $_____
% of Dollars Saved: _____%

Is there any revenue sharing between XYZ Contracted Administrator and the Case Management Company? _____Yes _____No.

If a revenue sharing exists what is the amount being shared? (An example might be the Case Management Fee is $125 / hour and the revenue sharing is $75 to Case Manager and $50 to XYZ Contracted Administrator). Please explain:

If sharing does exist is the any sharing with the Agent Broker or Consultant as compensation. If so please explain:

Please state whom fees/compensation is paid to:

Name:_____
Address:_____
City:_____ State:_____ Zip:_____
EIN or SSN:_____
Amount: $_____

Name:_____
Address:_____
City:_____ State:_____ Zip:_____
EIN or SSN:_____
Amount: $_____

Name:_____
Address:_____
City:_____ State:_____ Zip:_____
EIN or SSN:_____
Amount: $_____

PPO Network Contracted as PAR to the XXX Plan by the Contracted Administrator:

Please complete the appropriate table listed below: The *gross* is obtained from the Administrative Agreement as billed from the Contracted Administrator. The *net* is from the agreement and information requested from the PPO provider and/or Aggregator which includes the billing from the PPO.

PEPM Gross	Composite	Employee	EE + SP	EE+ 1	EE+Children	Family
Composite	$					
By Census		$	$	$	$	$

PEPM Net	Composite	Employee	EE + SP	EE+ 1	EE+Children	Family
Composite	$					
By Census		$	$	$	$	$

OR

% of Savings Gross	Composite	Employee	EE + SP	EE+ 1	EE+Children	Family
Composite	%					
By Census		%	%	%	%	%

% of Savings Net	Composite	Employee	EE + SP	EE+ 1	EE+Children	Family
Composite	%					
By Census		%	%	%	%	%

If there is a difference in the PEPM Gross and the PEPM Net, or % of Savings Gross and % of Savings Net, was the difference retained by the contracted administrator? _____Yes _____No.

If No then whom was the difference paid to?

Was this compensation disclosed or is this compensation considered undisclosed to the Fiduciaries of the Plan? Please Explain:

Is there a sharing of this compensation to the Agent, Broker or Consultant?

Please state whom fees/compensation is paid to:

Name:_____
Address:_____
City:_____ State:_____ Zip:_____
EIN or SSN:_____
Amount: $_____PEPM %_____ of savings

Name:_____
Address:_____
City:_____ State:_____ Zip:_____
EIN or SSN:_____
Amount: $_____PEPM %_____ of savings

Name:_____
Address:_____
City:_____ State:_____ Zip:_____
EIN or SSN:_____
Amount: $_____PEPM %_____ of savings

OON (Out of Network) Contracted as Non PAR to the XXX Plan by the Contracted Administrator:

Is there an aggregator contracted by XYZ Contracted Administrator? ____Yes ____No

As the Contracted Administrator, if not utilizing an Aggregator, are you providing the repricing "In House" utilizing PPO Agreements? ____ Yes ____No

As the Contracted Administrator, if not utilizing an Aggregator or utilization of a PPO Agreement, are you utilizing a % of Medicare or equivalent table? ____ Yes ____No

If yes please explain the table being utilized and the % being utilized. (As an example if utilizing Medicare is it based on a 125%? If utilizing a UCR what percentile is being utilized?

Please explain the methodologies used in the OON as either a repricing with PPO Contracts as a % or a PEPM Wrap, negotiation of fees, etc. as the structure used for XXX Plan.

Is the OON Based on a Wrap with a PEPM? _____ Yes _____ No

If a PPO network Wrap Please complete the PEPM Chart.

PEPM Gross	Composite	Employee	EE + SP	EE+ 1	EE+Children	Family
Composite	$					
By Census		$	$	$	$	$

PEPM Net	Composite	Employee	EE + SP	EE+ 1	EE+Children	Family
Composite	$					
By Census			$	$	$	$

And / OR

If Utilizing an Aggregator please complete the following:

% of Savings	Net by Aggregator	Gross charged By Contracted Administrator	Difference Gross Less Net
Charged	%	%	%

And / OR

If providing OON/Negotiation "In House" please complete the following: Is the amount charged based on the difference in the Gross Bill and the reduction applied whether utilizing a Medicare, UCR Table Etc. Please state table being utilized:

% of Savings	Net by Contracted Administrator	Gross charged By Contracted Administrator	Difference Gross Less Net
Charged	%	%	%

If there is a difference in the PEPM Gross and the PEPM Net, or % of Savings Gross and % of Savings Net, was the difference retained by the contracted administrator _____Yes _____No.

Was this compensation disclosed or is this compensation considered undisclosed to the Fiduciaries of the Plan. Please Explain:

Is there a sharing of this compensation to the Consultant, Agent and/or Broker as compensation?

Please state whom fees/compensation is paid to:

Name:_____
Address:_____
City:_____ State:_____ Zip:_____
EIN or SSN:_____
Amount: $_____PEPM %_____ of savings

Name:_____
Address:_____
City:_____ State:_____ Zip:_____
EIN or SSN:_____
Amount: $_____PEPM %_____ of savings

Name:_____
Address:_____
City:_____ State:_____ Zip:_____
EIN or SSN:_____
Amount: $_____PEPM %_____ of savings

Contracted PBM and Administrator

PBM Contracted to the XXX Plan by the Contracted Administrator:

The follow is the disclosure of any revenue sharing between the PBM, XYZ Administrator, Consultant, Broker or Agent. Due to the contract being executed with the XYZ Administrator, disclosure of all revenue whether sharing of administrative fees from PBM, addition of a PerScript Fee, Rebates and any other compensation paid by the PBM to the XYZ Administrator, Consultant, Broker or Agent.

Category	PBM	CA	ABC	Net Fees
Admin Fees				
PerScript Fee				
Reimbursement of Admin Fees				
Rebates				
Card Fees				
AWP Spread				
Dispensing Fee Spread				
Generic or Mac Spread				

Was this compensation disclosed or is this compensation considered undisclosed to the Fiduciaries of the Plan? Please Explain:

Is there a sharing of this compensation to the Consultant, Agent and or Broker as compensation?

Please state whom fees/compensation is paid to:

Name:_____
Address:_____
City:_____ State:_____ Zip:_____

EIN or SSN:_____
Amount: $_____PEPM   %_____ of savings

Name:_____
Address:_____
City:_____ State:_____ Zip:_____
EIN or SSN:_____
Amount: $_____PEPM   %_____ of savings

Name:_____
Address:_____
City:_____ State:_____ Zip:_____
EIN or SSN:_____
Amount: $_____PEPM   %_____ of savings

Contracted Stoploss and Administrator

Stoploss Contracted to the XXX Plan by the Contracted Administrator:

This is a request for disclosure of the compensation paid by the Stoploss Carrier and/or Managing General Underwriter to the XYZ Contracted Administrator and/or Consultant, Agent or Broker.

Stoploss Carrier and Underwriter:

Stoploss Carrier:_____
Managing General Underwriter:_____
Contact at MGU:_____ Phone:_____
Email:_____
Address:_____
City:_____ State:_____ Zip:_____
EIN or SSN:_____

Agent, Broker or Consultant of Record:

Firm Name:_____
Name:_____ Phone:_____
Email:_____
Address:_____
City:_____ State:_____ Zip:_____
EIN or SSN:_____

If Compensation is being Split Please indicate with whom by completing the following:

Firm Name:_____
Name:_____ Phone:_____
Email:_____
Address:_____
City:_____ State:_____ Zip:_____
EIN or SSN:_____
Percentage of Split: _____%

The rates for the Stoploss Agreement are as follow for XXX Plan:

Specific Contract	Specific Deductible	Effective Date	End Date	Specific Advance Y or N			
	$						
		Employee	EE + SP	EE+ 1	EE+Children	Family	
Initial Census							

Specific Contract used such as 12/12, 15/12, 12/15 etc.

Specific Gross Premium	Composite	Employee	EE + SP	EE+ 1	EE+Children	Family
Composite	$					
By Census		$	$	$	$	$

Specific Net Premium	Composite	Employee	EE + SP	EE+ 1	EE+Children	Family
Composite	$					
By Census		$	$	$	$	$

And/Or

Aggregate Contract	Minimum Attachment Point	Effective Date	End Date	Aggregate Accommodation Y or N		
	$					
		Employee	EE + SP	EE+ 1	EE+Children	Family
Initial Census						
Funding Factors		$	$	$	$	$

Aggregate Contract used such as 12/12, 15/12, 12/15 etc.

Aggregate Gross Premium	Composite	Employee	EE + SP	EE+ 1	EE+Children	Family
Composite	$					
Census		$	$	$	$	$

AggregateNet Premium	Composite	Employee	EE + SP	EE+ 1	EE+Children	Family
Composite	$					
Census		$	$	$	$	$

Aggregate Accommodation Fee:

Is a fee for Aggregate Accommodation being paid? _____Yes _____No If yes, what is the fee on a PEPM Basis charged by the Stoploss or MGU? $_____

Has any markup in the fee be done and charged to XXX Plan? _____
Yes _____No
If Yes, what is the fee with the markup included on a PEPM Basis: $_____
Was this disclosed to XXX Plan Fiduciaries in writing? _____Yes _____No

Additional Compensation from Stoploss Carrier and/or MGU:

In addition to the commission for the Stoploss contract above, is there any revenue being paid to the Contracted Administrator as an override, bonus or any other basis for compensation from Stoploss Carrier and/or Managing General Underwriter to Contracted Administrator and/or Agent Broker or Consultant? ____Yes ____No

If Yes, then describe the compensation arrangement/agreement:

Forensic Decision Mapping

Forensic Decision Mapping provides a structured approach in deciphering the objective facts and data. The Forensic Decision Mapping is broken down into six sections.

1. subject of the issue
2. definition of the issue
3. forensic/analytic basis for decision necessity
4. impact on strategy
5. decision mapping
6. notes.

The Forensic Decision Mapping provides a process for finding the objective facts on the issue(s) at hand. Many times, there will be additional areas that are related to the issue at hand for investigation. These additional areas should have additional Forensic Decision Mappings to provide a structure for the investigation. Utilizing these formats provides a basis to explain the process used for the Forensic Investigation in a logical based format to be used when explaining the process to the hiring entity with subsequent documentation from the objective facts obtained. It is important to note that this work is discoverable if a litigation is filed. This discovery will show the Forensic Investigator utilized a logical process for uncovering the objective facts. In addition, if the Forensic Investigator is required to testify either by deposition or in court it provides a basis to investigative process with documentation received and analyzed for the objective facts pertaining to the issue(s) at hand. This creates simplicity when questioned in a deposition or explaining to the jury in court. The logical process is better understood when presented in the Matrix of the Forensic Decision Mapping, the information requested, the process of the information and the objective findings. This structure can and should be used if required to provide a report to the hiring entity or the court of law.

As the Forensic Investigator, it is not your job to determine innocence or guilt as that is left to the legal process. The job of the Forensic Investigator is to provide the objective facts that pertain to the issue at hand. The Forensic Decision Mapping structure will help the Forensic Investigator to best present the facts in court and when under cross examination.

Code of Ethics: "ACFEI and its members are to remain completely objective and use their ability to serve justice by making an accurate determination of the facts involved." *(American College of Forensic Examiners Principles of Professional Practice)*

The following is extracted from a case in regard to Stoploss reimbursements on both the specific Stoploss and aggregate Stoploss.

Subject is where the concentration is based on complaint, such as: 2009 Stoploss Reimbursements and the entities with whom the issue encompasses on the vendor level.

Subject: 2009 Stoploss Reimbursements	Contracted Administrator and Carrier Underwriting Managers via Insurance Stoploss Carrier

Definition of the issue is stating what data issues are sought and the entities involved. An example:

Definition of Issue:	Validation of Specific and Aggregate filings were made with all funds

being transferred to Plan Sponsor also known as Plan Sponsor Health Plan from Contracted
Administrator and Carrier Underwriting Insurance Stoploss Carrier on policy 40-19-042
for Stoploss contract period Jan 1, 2009 though Dec 31, 2009.

Forensic/Analytic basis for decision necessity defines why the decision is necessary. Example:

Forensic/Analytic basis for decision necessity:
Validation of accounting of all deposits, claims and vendor payments. Validation of all filings
made from TPA to Carrier Underwriting Managers for both Specific and Aggregate filings.

Impact on Strategy puts in perspective what is being validated, analyzed or verified. There are usually three impacts on strategy statements made. When going beyond three impact statements, a second decision mapping is suggested. Example:

Impact on Strategy		
Item 1: TPA validation of check registers, Specific Claims, Aggregate Claims were made and funds transmitted to Plan Sponsor.	**Item 2:** Carrier - processed all filings for Specific and Aggregate claims. Copies of all claims filed from TPA with checks written for reimbursement to Plan Sponsor	**Item 3:** Validation of all Specific and aggregate payments received and full account of all transactions via check registers received from TPA and correspondence.

Once this information is compiled, then map out the flow.

Forensic Decision Mapping provides a logical structured sequence in which to review the objective data for validation or invalidation of the issues at hand. The following is a structured example from the case information listed above.

Stoploss Reimbursements

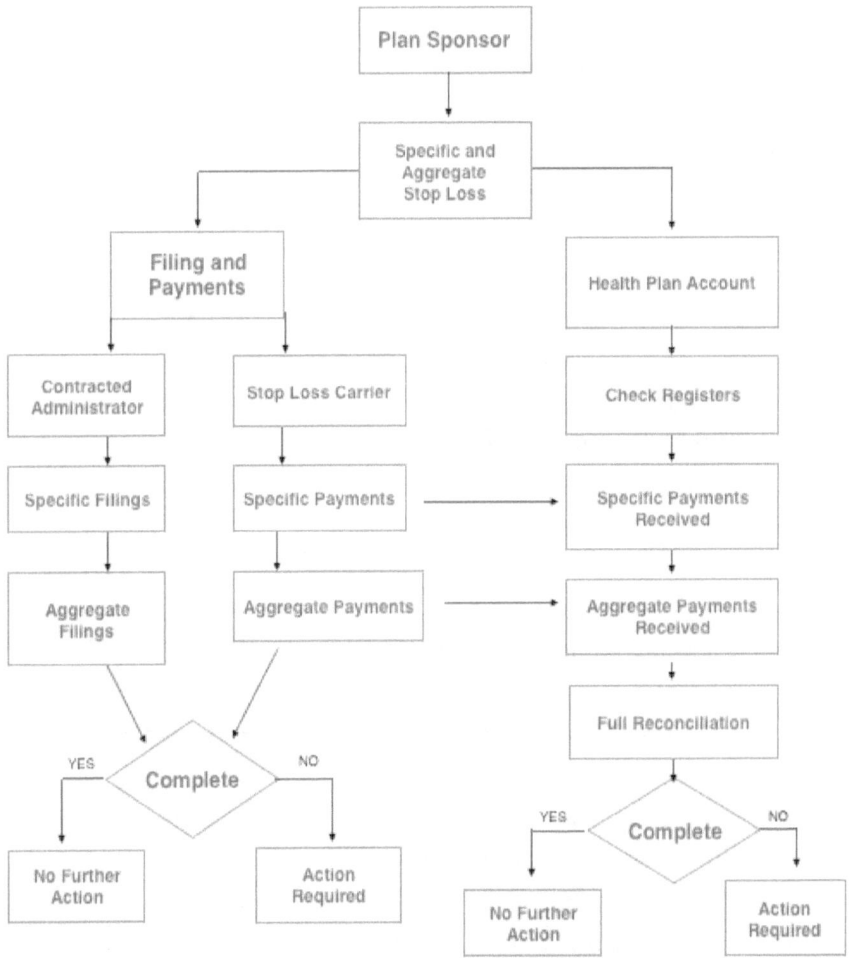

The logical structure provides the validation or invalidation of the facts at hand. This decision mapping also provides the comparative analytic structure for verification from the specific areas at issue for validation of the money, the depositing and tracking funds to the Plan Health Benefit Account.

Notes provide a multifaceted approach as to the information that will be needed and the corresponding findings of fact(s). The following was a preliminary note listing information needed as well as other issues from other data previously analyzed and compared as probabilities for validation on other data.

1. **Information needed from Plan Sponsor:** Bank Statements 2009 Plan Year. All check
2. registers received from TPA. All copies of Specific and Aggregate Reimbursements received.
3. Copy of Stoploss contract issued by Carrier via Insurance Policy 40-19-042. Copy of
4. Administrative Service Agreement from Contracted Administrator. Copies of checks from July 2009
5. through December 31, 2009 with endorsements.
6. **Information needed from Carrier:** Copy of Stoploss contract via Insurance 40-19-0442.
7. Copies of all Specific and Aggregate filings from TPA for Transit System with all correspondence.
8. Copies of all Specific and Aggregate reimbursements paid with copies of front and back of checks.
9.
10. **Information from TPA:** Copy of full check register for PY 2009 (Jan 1, 2009 through Dec 31, 2009
11. Copy of 75% Specific Report as well as Aggregate Report. After information is received from
12. Plan Sponsor and Carrier, additional information: LAG Report, Detailed Claims Report, copies of all
13. filings submitted to Carrier for Specific and Aggregate Reimbursement requests with
14. Correspondence.
15. Based on preliminary findings an additional request to PBM on all Rx claims billed to
16. Plan Sponsor for 2009 PY with copies of checks issued for payment. Copies of all audited Rx
17. **Claims from PBM Auditing Co:** with invoices and checks received as payments from Plan

18. Sponsor. An additional comparison of the billing and payments made to PBM vs audited results
19. from PBM Auditing Co.
20. Probability exists that TPA did not process the audited Rx claims but instead just paid PBM
21. on the billings issued. PBM Auditing Co. appears to have been paid from Plan Sponsor for
22. auditing which was not processed by Contracted Administrator, creating a higher liability for the
23. health plan. Differences to be determined from reports analyzed.
24. **Information from PBM:** Copies of Rebate Checks issued to Plan Sponsor for the 2009 Plan
25. Year.

Two additional Forensic Decision Mappings were appropriate for the validation and analysis of the PBM, PBM Auditing Company, Contracted Administrator as an expansion for validating the objective facts. From the agreements reviewed for the Plan Sponsor, there was a contractual agreement for Prospective PBM Auditing. This brought up the basis to determine thereview to validate the propective audited results were processed by the Contracted Administrator for the Plan Sponsors Health Plan for reduction of cost for the prescriptions in the health plan. The first deals with the PBM (Prescription Benefit Management) company and the second deals with the PBM Auditing Company.

The following are the Forensic Decision Mappings for these issues.

PBM Provider

Subject: PBM Provider	PBM for Rx
Definition of Issue:	Validation of Rx claims processed by PBM Rx with dates of

transmittal of billings and verification of dates and amounts paid for Plan Sponsor.
Forensic/Analytic basis for decision necessity:
Validation of Rx claims processed by PBM Rx with dates of transmittal and validation of paid amounts
per report of American Administrators for Plan Sponsor.

Impact on Strategy		
Item 1: Validation of amounts in	**Item 2:** Verification of amounts	**Item 3:** Discrepancy in Contracted
billing vs dates remitted for	paid per participant for inclusion in	Administrator reports
payment by Contracted	specific and aggregate for Plan	vs PBM Rx billings and dates
Administrator for PS Plan.	Sponsors Health Plan.	incurred vs paid for inclusion in
		Specific and aggregate for Plan.

PBM Provider submitted claims in both an electronic version and paper format for processing the detailed billing. It is important to review the documentation and procedures used in setting the format of the Forensic Decision Mapping.

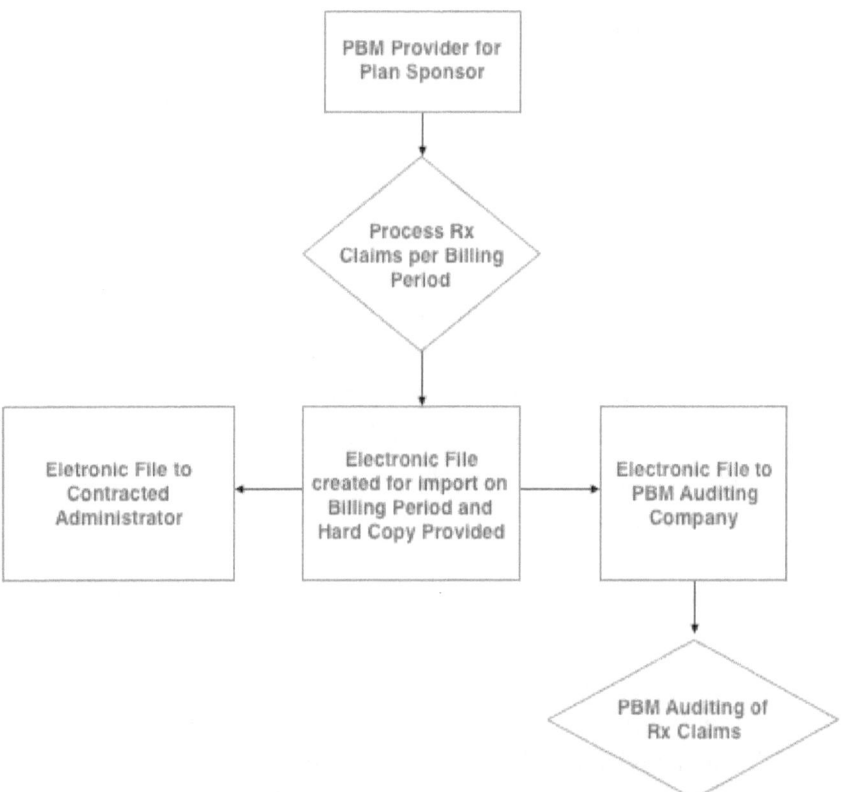

PBM Rx was contracted to provide PBM Services for the Plan Sponsors Health Plan. The requested from PBM Rx is for validation of the Rx Benefit for the participants of Plan Sponsors Health Plan. The information requested will provide a valid claims base and timing of billing to the Health Plan and utilized for verification of the reports issued by Contracted Administrator.

The Stoploss contract with the Carrier was a 12/12 specific and aggregate contract. The requested and the analytics and forensics which are applied will show the timing of the billing and remittance information of payments to apply against the parameters of the 12/12 incurred and paid basis of the Carriers contract for inclusion in the filing periods for both specific and aggregate since both have the inclusion of Rx as a factor for eligible claims.

Information needed from PBM Rx.

1. Copies of all billings for the Plan Sponsors Health Plan by billing cycle. These reports should be in an .xls format as well as a .pdf. If the fee billing for administration from PBM Rx invoice is in a word document then it should be provided.
2. Copies of all payments received by PBM Rx on the Plan Sponsors Health Plan with the amounts of remittance, the billing cycle it is applied to and the dates received by PBM Rx
3. Copies of all executed agreements for the Rx Plan - including the contract between PBM Rx and Plan Sponsor. This information should include the work sheets used in setting up the plan for the Plan Sponsor

The information above will be compiled and compared to the reports from Contracted Administrator, Check registers for payments provided by Contracted Administrator and timing of payments for inclusion of the Stoploss Agreement with Spectrum Underwriters for validation of the 12/12 incurred and paid base. Check registers sent to Plan Sponsor from Contracted Administrator will be analyzed for release of payments for timing issues and inclusion in the Stoploss Agreement.

The information received will be used in comparison of the Audited reports from PBM Auditing Company for Calculation purposes as well. for the 2009 Plan Year for Plan Sponsors Health Plan.

Amount of rebate should be used to reduce the calculated Prescription (Rx) claims for Plan Sponsor Health Plan for Plan Year 2009. Not applying Rx rebates increases cost and exposure to the plan.

PBM Auditing

Subject: PBM Auditing	PBM Auditing Company
Definition of Issue:	Review the Rx auditing of the plan and use of Prospective audit in the
	processing of the Rx claims. Compare and contrast the billing per cycle transmitted by PBM Rx to
	Contracted Administrator and that of the audited Rx transmitted by PBM Auditing Company. to
	Contracted Administrator for processing on the Plan Sponsors Health Plan.
Forensic/Analytic basis for decision necessity:	
Review the Aggregate Excess Report from Contracted Administrator for PY 2009. Compare the	
Prescription claims posted in the report to the PBM audited billings.	
Impact on Strategy	

Item 1: Non use of audited Rx by PBM audit potential affect on RX claims. Audit use may have affect in decreasing exposure to Plan Sponsor.	Item 2: PBM audit contracted for plan and paid by Plan Sponsors from Medical Plan Account for services and audit reports.	Item 3: Validate Contracted Administrators use or non use of audit per billing period on Plan Sponsor Rx Benefit.

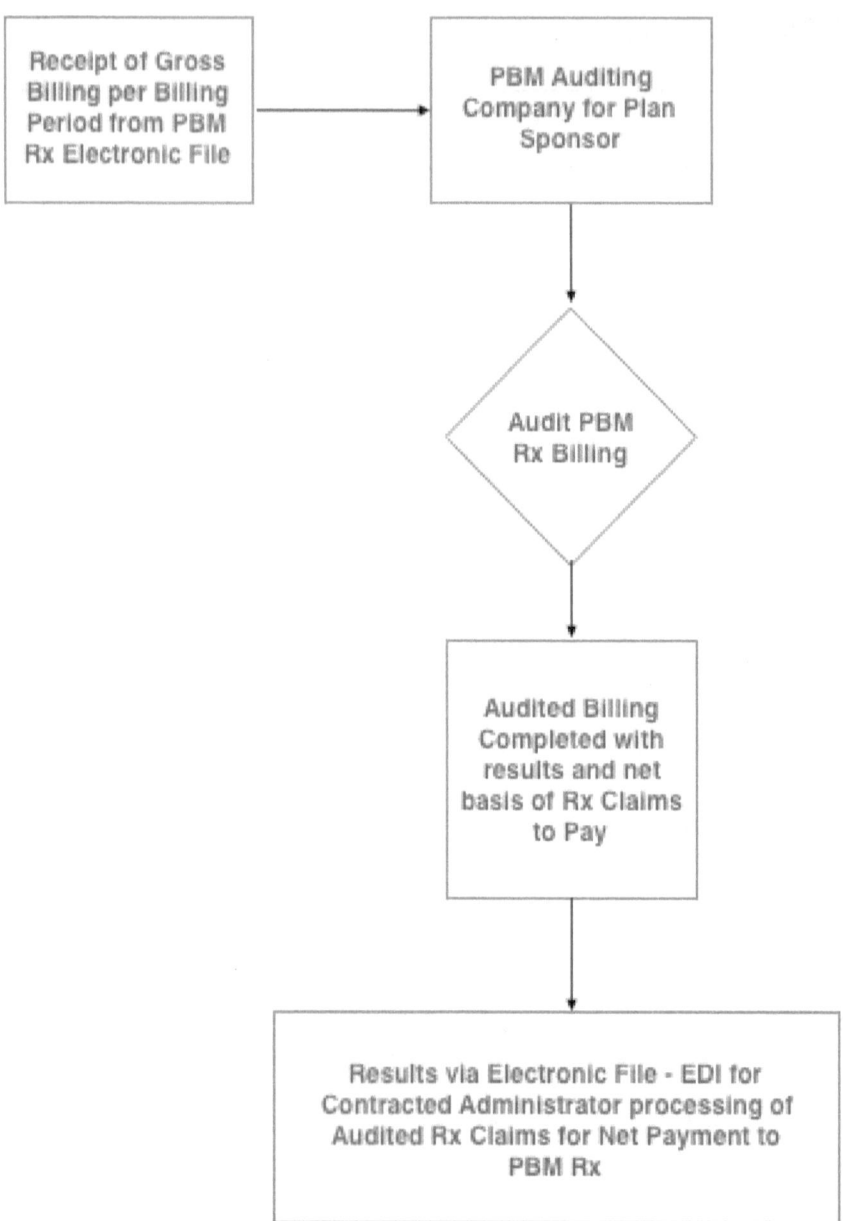

PBM Auditor. was contracted to the Plan Sponsors Health Plan for auditing on a prospective basis the billing from PBM Rx. The audited results were to be processed and the net cost of the audited bill to be sent with a check to PBM Rx for the billing of that period. PBM Rx would have the opportunity to challenge the audit. This challenge would be between PBM Rx and PBM Auditing Company The results of the challenge could be upheld on the audit or a requirement to cut an additional check from the challenge only on those claims that the challenge overturned the specific claims in question on the audit.

Information Request to complete Forensics and Analytics.

1. Copies of all audited Rx on Plan Sponsor for 2009 Plan Year from PBM Auditing Company. these reports will need to be provided in both a .xls and .pdf format. If a word document accompanied the audit reports for each billing period audited then the document must accompany the specific billing period audited.
2. Copies of all invoices for services sent from PBM Auditing Co. to Contracted Administrator on behalf of Plan Sponsor In addition, payments received from the Plan Sponsors Health Plan with the check number, amount and date of check received and the invoice it pertained to.
3. Copy of executed agreement(s) between PBM Auditing Co., Plan Sponsor and Contracted Administrator. This includes the service agreement and cost of services for PBM Auditing to Plan Sponsors Health Plan and any NDA (Non Disclosure Agreements) signed by the parties PBM Auditing Co., Plan Sponsor and Contracted Administrator.
4. Copies of all documentation provided by Plan Sponsor, Contracted Administrator and PBM Rx used in the setup, and auditing of the Rx claims for Plan Sponsor.
5. Provide a flow on how PBM Auditing Co. received the claims per billing cycle from PBM Rx. The processing of the claims being audited and the transmittal of the claims to Contracted Administrator for processing. Be specific - if audited claims were transmitted to Contracted Administrator via SFTP with a key, state so.

The requested information above will be analyzed against the information disclosed in the Contracted Administrator report to Plan Sponsor on the Aggregate Risk Report for Plan Year 1/1/09 - 12/31/09. The dates of the audited Rx billing transmissions on the date posted to the secure site for Contracted Administrator to pick up and process will also be compared to the claims by month listed in the report.

The check registers from Plan Sponsor are also requested for the 2009 plan year in total. The registers sent to Plan Sponsor from Contracted Administrator for approval to release the payment of RX claims processed. This information will be applied to the proper billing cycles for timing of Rx claim payments as well as which billing reports were processed for payments - PBM Rx gross Rx billing per billing cycle or PBMAuditing Co. audited Rx Billing per cycle. In addition, the check registers will validate the payments for services to PBM Auditing Co. for PBM auditing on a prospective basis.

If you suspect something, state it. The objective facts will either prove or disprove the suspicion. Look closely for validation either positive or negative.

Plan Sponsor

Subject: Plan Sponsor	Plan Sponsor
Definition of Issue:	Claims processed, Information for 5500 PY 2009, Accuracy of Reports
received from Contracted Administrator (TPA). Any issues known by Plan Sponsor from	
TPA on internal problems which could have affected claims processing.	
Forensic/Analytic basis for decision necessity:	
Review of 5500 PY 2009 for accuracy, reports from TPA to Plan Sponsor, Separate calculation independent of	

TPA based on fees, premiums, claims paid by plan. Review of Plan Bank Account for duplications of claims paid, rebates received from PBM and refunds from providers for overpayment or duplicate payments.

Impact on Strategy		
Item 1: Review of information	**Item 2:** Review of check registers	**Item 3:** Determination of Agent of
on reports for accuracy and	approved, receipt of rebates PBM	Record as perceived from Plan
inclusion on 5500 Form PY 2009	or refunds applied back to medical	Sponsor.
Including Aggregate Filing by TPA	plan account.	

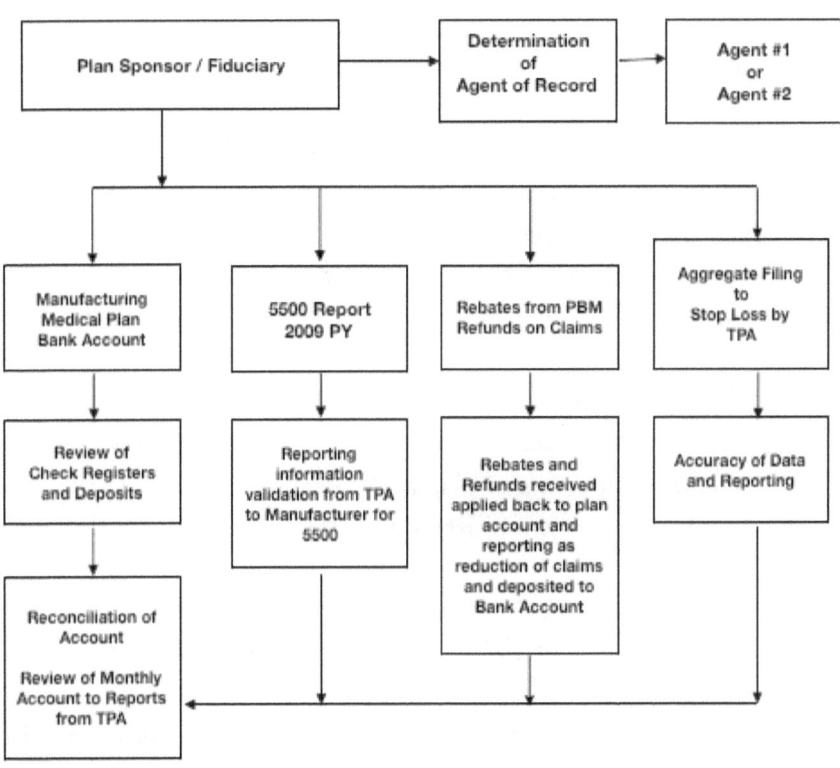

Plan Sponsor and Fiduciary for the Self Funded Plan.

A complete review of the Plan Sponsor Medical Plan Bank Account is warented for the accuracy of the claims processed and paid in accordance with the Stoploss Agreement of the Plan.

Information needed

1. Check Registers provided from Contracted Administrator to Plan Sponsor and approved by Plan Sponsor to Contracted Administrator.
2. Monthly Bank Statements from Plan Sponsors on Bank Account. Validation of claims paid per month vs check registers from TPA. Deposits made for account.
3. Reports issued fromContracted Administrator to Plan Sponsor monthly.
4. Rebates received by Plan Sponsor from PBM Rx for PY 2009 with date of check and amount. Validation of depositing to account and reduction of cost of claims.
5. Refunds from providers for overpayment and duplicate payments for plan. Validation of depositing to account and reduction of claims reported.
6. Copies of monthly billing from TPA to Plan Sponsor.
7. Copy of 2009 5500 Form with Schedules A and C for validation of correct reporting of plan and costs.
8. Validation of Agent of Record from Plan Sponsor for Plan.
9. Copies of all agreements with vendors to the plan.
10. Copy of filing to Stoploss Carrier from TPA on request for reimbursement of claims exceeding the Specific Stoploss and or Aggregate Stoploss.
11. Contracted Administrator disclosure of any problems in processing of claims as conveyed to Plan Sponsor.

The information above once received will be compiled and processed to establish the accuracy of claims costs, vendors paid, providers paid,

Stoploss paid, compensation paid. This will be utilized in a comparison to reported vs actual costs to validate the claims paid, vendors paid, compensation paid.

Validation has been received on the rebates paid to LBC from HealthSmart Rx. Check # 2129 for $16,105.25 issued on October 14, 2010 to Plan Sponsor and mailed to the attention of Plan Sponsor Representative for Qtr 1 2009: $3,864.00, Qtr 2 2009: $4,224.50, Qtr 3 2009: 3,949.75 and Qtr. 4 2009: $4,067.00 were validated by email from PBM Rx Representative email October 1, 2012.

Contracted Administrator

Subject: TPA / ASO	Contracted Administrators	
Definition of Issue:	Accuracy of processing of claims. Validation of reports submitted	
to Plan Sponsor as well as the submission of the Aggregate Filing to Stoploss Underwriter for		
reimbursement of claims for the 2009 PY.		
Forensic/Analytic basis for decision necessity:		
Review of all claims, calculation and analysis.		
Impact on Strategy		
Item 1: Errors in processing due to corporate decisions.	Item 2: Potential lack of accuracy in reporting and compilation of data.	Item 3: Not processing claims from audits done example PBM Audits.

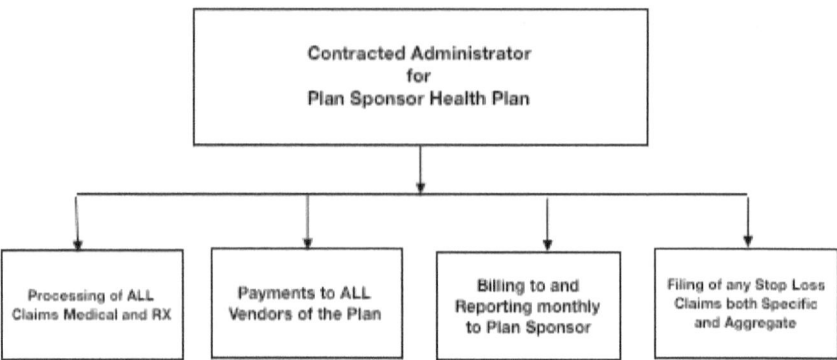

Contracted Administrator was the contracted Third Party Administrator for the Plan Sponsor Health Plan. Contracted Administrator was responsible for all claims processing, reporting, compliance, and coordination with all vendors involved in the plan. Contracted Administrator utilized the Administration System for Administration of the Plan. The reports requested are from the Administration System.

Review of all vendors, claims (Medical and Rx), processing of all claims on a timely basis, accuracy of claims processed and reporting.

Information Requested to perform Forensics and Analytics.

1. Detailed Medical Claim Report for the Plan Year 2009. The report in the Administration System is called **Employee/Dependent Claims Analysis.** This report should include both medical and prescription claims. This report should be requested in a .xls and .pdf format.
2. **Claims Lag Report** for the Plan Year January 1, 2009 through December 31, 2009. The flag on this report should be set with the incurred date. This report should be requested in a .xls and .pdf format.
3. **Employee / Dependent Claims Analysis** for January 1, 2009 through December 31, 2009 and using only the Expense Employee. This is normally set up as **Employee #1**. This report should provide a report on All vendors to the plan with check

numbers and amounts with date paid. This report will not include Benjamin Byrne & Associates as this compensation was processed from Contracted Administrator directly with Agent #2. This report should be requested in a .xls and .pdf format.

4. **Group Aggregate Report** for January 1, 2009 through December 31, 2009. This needs to be requested the Master Group for Plan Sponsor which will include all sub groups under the Master Group and Locations / Divisions. This should be shown by month in the report. This report should be requested in a .xls and .pdf format.

5. **Check Register Report** for January 1, 2009 through December 31, 2009. Needs to be requested on Master Group which should include all Locations / Divisions. This report should be requested in a .xls and .pdf format.

6. Copies of transmittal check registers sent to Plan Sponsor with email and the emails from Plan Sponsor release of the checks from January 1, 2009 through December 31, 2009.

7. Copies of Subrogation Claims filed for the plan with specific information including, Letters filed, amounts received for the plan, costs incurred. Validation of any amounts received were applied back to the plan and provided to Plan Sponsor for deposit into the Health Plan Account.

8. Copies of any checks received by providers for over payments, duplicate payments, Verification of the refunds sent to Plan Sponsor for deposit into their Health Plan Account.

Representative, President of Contracted Administrator - problems for the Satellite Office.

An internal problem arose with Contracted Administrator on April 1, 2009. This problem came about with the transfer of the software and data to off site computer cloud company the evening of March 31, 2009. This transfer took place at the direction of the President Representative. There were no contingency plans. Contracted Administrator was not able to edit, adjudicate nor write a payment to a vendor due to a software issue that occurred during this transfer. This went on for about 23 days. On the 23rd day at approximately 4:30 Administration put a senior Analyst on this issue and the problem was corrected.

A second issue was found in the filter for duplicate claims which was found by the Senior Claims Administrator which found the filter that throws out the duplicate claims had been changed in a training session. This problem allowed claims to be processed and paid that were duplicates.

A third issue occurred with a vendor for processing the Rx via EDI with the system. This issue was between Contracted Administrator President and the programmer Contracted Programmer on payment of services. Contracted Programmer shut the program off and issues on processing arose with delays.

From these circumstances creates the question of the accuracy of the administration and processing of claims.

Medical claims may have had the discounts denied due to the delays in processing by the providers contracted by the PPO Network.

Some providers may have received duplicate payments which were not followed up on by the American Administrator staff and possibly depended on the providers to be honest and return the duplicate payments.

The medical and Rx claims came in EDI for processing for Plan Sponsor Due to the problems mentioned above a detailed analytical view of the administration, claims and accuracy are questioned and possibly would warrant a full reprocessing of all claims to validate accuracy.

The findings above lead to additional investigation structure(s) for Forensic Decision Mapping. These specific areas will lead to several additional Forensic Decision Mappings to provide a structure for reviewing the information in order to extract the objective facts pertaining to the Impact on Strategy. Investigation and interviews from employees at the contracted administrator provide findings with regard to problems at the Contracted Administrator.

Aggregator

Subject: Aggregator	Aggregator Company
Definition of Issue:	Validation of PPO billing, PAR Claims, Non Par Claims processed for
discounts and applied to the Plan Sponsor Health Plan for PY 2009.	
Forensic/Analytic basis for decision necessity:	
Proper allocation of claims and discounts processed for the plan and validation against reports and	
Information provided by Contracted Administrator.	
Impact on Strategy		
Item 1: Validation of Par claims	Item 2: Validation of Non-Par /	Item 3: Validation of billing for
with discounts for processing by	negotiated claims with reductions	PPO (PAR) access and Non-PAR/
Contracted Administrator.	for processing by Contracted	Negotiated claims with reductions
	Administrator.	

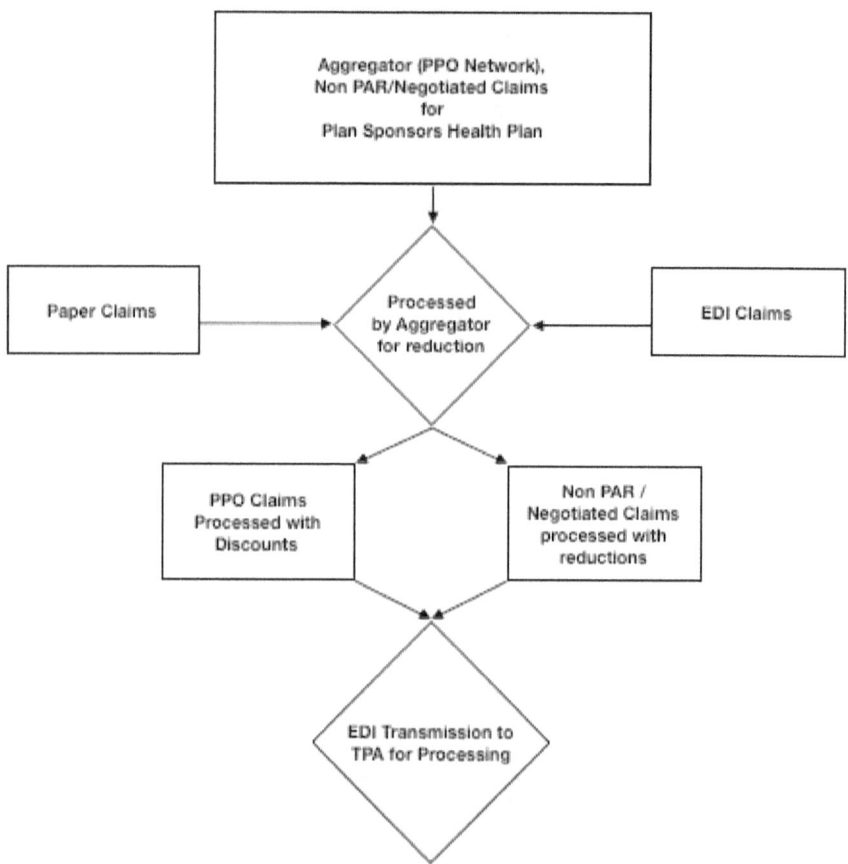

Aggregator Company was contracted for the Plan to provide PPO (PAR) processing and access and Non-PAR / Negotiation for claims outside of PPO (PAR). Aggregator Company received claims in paper or EDI from providers to the Plan Sponsor Health Plan for 2009. Claims were scanned, OCR conversion and discounts applied. Information was transmitted to Contracted Administrator via secure EDI file through sftp protocol. Contracted Administrator imported file to Administration Software System, processed eligibility claims via the adjudication protocols set up in the system base on the plan design and the plan the participant participated in.

This service is contracted by Contracted Administrator for the Plan Sponsor Health Plan for the 2009 PY.

Information needed from Aggregator Company

1. Validation of the PPO Access Fees charged to Contracted Administrator and payments received from TPA.
2. Validation of the PPO Access Fees charged to Contracted Administrator and payments received from TPA.
3. Validation of the % of savings charged for Non-PAR and Negotiated Claims with Contracted Administrator.
4. Validation of the % savings cost charged to Contracted Administrator and payments received from TPA.
5. Copy of all EDI files transmitted for Contracted Administrator processing of claims for Plan Sponsor Health Plan for the 2009 PY.

This information is to be used for validation of when claims were available to Contracted Administrator for processing to verify timing of processing. Additionally, the discounts actually processed by Aggregator Company for claim reduction and validation of claims by month as compared to the totals reported by Contracted Administrator.

This information will show if discounts were lost by Contracted Administrator for time delays in processing the claims for the Plan Sponsor Health Plan for PY 2009. This will also show the if all claims were processed timely for inclusion in the Stoploss Agreement on a 12/12 basis.

A specific process will need to be done with an out side TPA or utilizing the services of Administration Software in the duplication of the set up of the plans, import of individuals to the plan(s) with all dates of plan entries, changes for those who may have elected COBRA, all rates for all vendor fees to the plan, Stop Loss premiums, funding factors, Parameters for Stoploss contract on a specific and aggregate basis etc. The reprocessing of all claims by date and validated via independent processing will validate or invalidate the totals as reported by Contracted

Administrator for the Specific or Aggregate eligible claims submitted to Stoploss Company.

Managed Care

Subject: Managed Care	Managed Care Company
Definition of Issue:	Validation of billing for UR/Precert and Case Management for the
Plan Sponsors Health Plan PY 2014.	
Forensic/Analytic basis for decision necessity:	
Validation of the billing processed by Contracted Administrator for the Plan Sponsors	
Health Plan for PY 2014.	

Impact on Strategy		
Item 1: UR/PreCert billing	**Item 2:** Verification of Case	**Item 3:**
verification for 2014 PY	Management Billing for PY 2014	
	for inclusion in claims.	

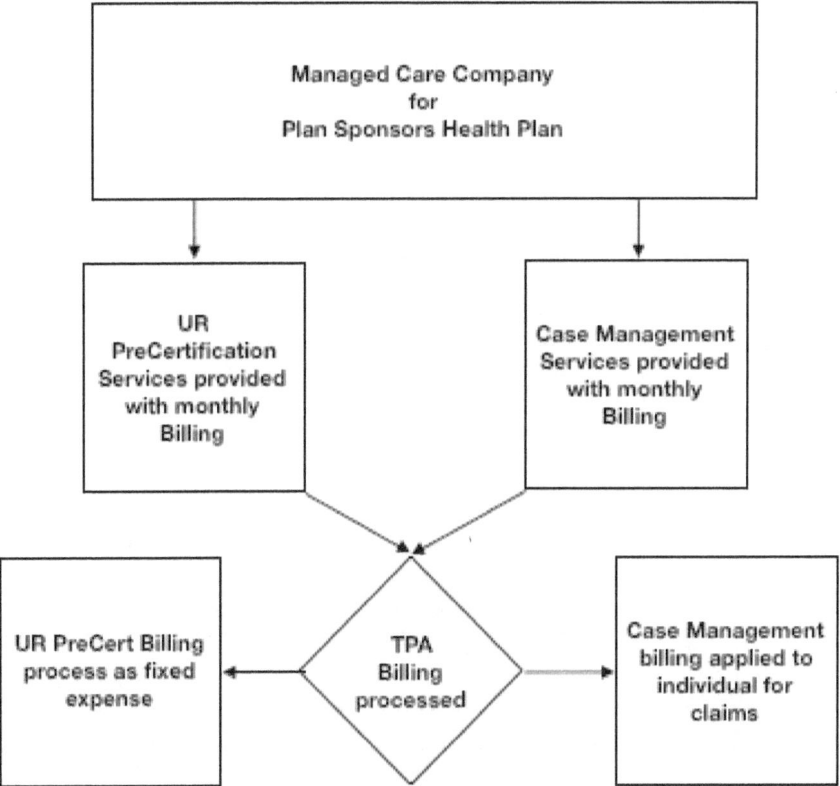

Managed Care Company was contracted to provide UR/PreCert and Case Management to the Plan Sponsors Health Plan for the 2014 PY

Information needed from Managed Care Company

1. Copy of Agreement for service to thePlan Sponsors. Health Plan for the PY 2014. This information will verify the charges made for UR/PreCert on a PEPM basis and the hourly rate charged for Case Management.
2. Copies of billings to Contracted Administrator for UR/PreCert and Case Management and copies of checks as payments received by Managed Care Company for the Plan Sponsors Health Plan for PY 2014.

This information will be compiled and compared to the information received from Contracted Administrator and Plan Sponsors records received for accuracy.

The information on the Case Management billing will be processed to the claims by individual provided with with Case Management for calculation of accuracy of processing and validation of any Specific Claims and Aggregate Claims applied on contract with Stoploss Company.

Accounting

Subject: Accounting	Review and reconcile Health Benefit Plan Account for PY 2015 Plan Sponsors Health Benefit Plan	
Definition of Issue:	Process all check register placing information into the right categories	
for validation of the account and accuracy of the balance.		
Forensic/Analytic basis for decision necessity:		
Review all transactions by category to validate the vendors to the plan and accuracy of reporting of fact.		
Impact on Strategy		
Item 1: View each category of the plan for accuracy.	Item 2: Establishment of cost of actual plan	Item 3: Utilize information in providing accuracy of comparative
		forensic analysis on each area of
		the plan.

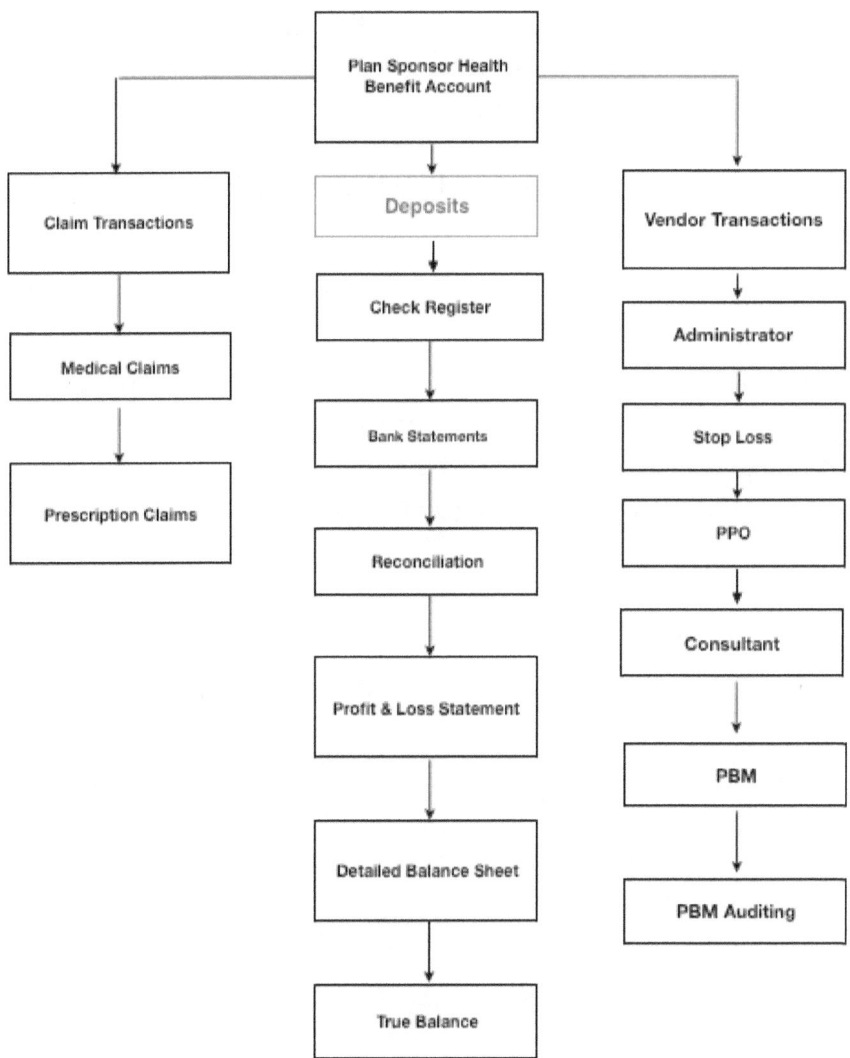

The accounting is a very important part of validating the transactions and using this information in the comparative analytics when viewing the various transactions and validating the information received. These transactions are compared to the contractual agreements in the self funded health plan.

The following chapter discuss structure of the accounts and accounting. Depending on the definition of the issue at hand, the accounting can be a very valuable objective base.

Extracting the information provides a basis for validating each area in the Chart of Accounts.

Summary

The Forensic Decision Mapping is designed to provide a process for finding the objective facts on the issue(s) at hand. The Forensic Decision Mapping is designed to be flexible to encompass the various issues which has an effect on obtaining and analyzing the objective facts.

Accounting and Accounts

In the initial area of concern the Plan Sponsor may make a statement, "The funds just do not add up from the reports we are receiving to the amount of funds we should have."

This statement should provide the investigator areas of examination. The areas for examination should include but not be limited to a financial investigation on the funds. Documentation should be requested from the Plan Sponsor and Contracted Administrator to provide clarification and comparison of the transactions.

Documentation from the Plan Sponsor should include the following for each of the plan years in question:

1. A written statement for the concern, the banking structure used, ownership of the banking relationship (account), the process of funding the account, the process with the Contracted Administrator for payment to the providers and vendors to the plan.
2. A copy of the bank account information, monthly statements, reconciliation done on the account from the plan sponsor.
3. A copy of the reports received from the Contracted Administrator for the written statement of concern.
4. A copy of the Administrative Service Agreement and contractual agreements with all vendors to the plan.

5. A copy of the Plan Document.
6. Copies of quotes for the plan.
7. Copies of correspondence between the Plan Sponsor and Contracted Administrator on the area of concern.
8. Copies of all detailed invoices to the Plan Sponsor.
9. Copies of all reports from the Contracted Administrator.
10. Copies of all check registers submitted to the Plan Sponsor from the Contracted Administrator.

Documentation from the Contracted Administrator should include the following:

1. Statement of process for the funding of the claims account, transmission of check registers and how this is to work (in their own words).
2. Copies of quotes for each of the plan years in question.
3. Copy of the Administrative Service Agreement and all vendor agreements.
4. Copy of the Plan Document.
5. Copy of the Banking Arrangement and documentation with the bank on the account ownership. (This is an important detail. Some Contracted Administrators will have the account set up under their company and state they break out the funds internally for each client with their production software. This is a basis for commingling of funds or it may be stated they set the account up as an FBO for the client which should allow for bank statements to be produced).
6. Copies of all bank statements for the plan for each of the plan years in question.
7. Copies of detailed check registers for each processing date transmitted to the Plan Sponsor for each of the plan years in question.
8. Copies of all detailed monthly invoices for the plan for each of the plan years in question.

9. Copy of the Aggregate Report for each of the plan years in question.
10. Copies of the 50% specific reporting by month for each of the plan years in question.

Timeline Documentation

Once the information is received it is important to establish the timeline of events. This timeline will be valuable as a reference for the investigator as well as the hiring entity. The timeline structure is a preference for the investigator by using a linear format of a chronological format. At times, both structures may be used. Examples of the timelines are illustrated below.

Linear Timeline

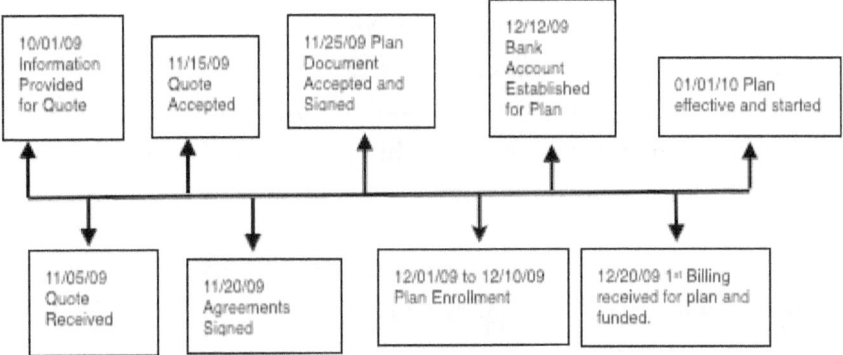

Chronological Time Line

10/01/2009 - Agent asked to quote medical plan. Information is provided to the agent.

11/05/2009 - Agent presents quote for the upcoming plan year 01/01/2010.

11/15/2009 - Quote is accepted and agent informed.

11/20/2009 - Agent presents Agreements to be signed. Agreements signed.

11/25/2009 - Agent presents Plan Document. Plan Document accepted and Signed.
12/01/2009 to 12/10/20009 - Enrollment by agent of employees for participation in plan.
12/12/2009 - Bank Account established for Plan.
12/20/2009 - Received first billing for the plan starting 01/01/2010 and amounts is deposited in account.
01/01/2010 - Plan Starts.

With the chronological timeline the investigator can state as much detail as needed.

It is important for the Plan to have its own account. The account should be in the Plan name and set up at the bank of choice from the Plan Sponsor. This is due to the ownership of the dollars utilized for the plan, and provides a full accounting and accountability of the Plan's finances.

There are instances where under ERISA Plan and Non ERISA Plan structures the ASO (Insurance Company) and / or TPAs (Third Party Administrators) will have the Plan Sponsor transfer funds for the Plan to them via wire or other method. This process should throw up a red flag for the Forensic Investigator.

There is a caution to this structure as these funds may now be deemed to be the ownership of the ASO or TPA.

Account Structures

In the proper utilization of the account the ASO (Insurance Company) or TPA (Third Party Administrator) should only have a signature authority on the account for issuance of payments for claims.

When disclosed and non disclosed compensation is discussed in the following examples, this will also apply to the Agents, Brokers and Consultants. There may have been negotiations between the entities in regard to compensation for use of their services. If using the New

Matrix, this should not be an issue as the Plan Sponsor will own the contracts for the Plan on a net basis. The following are examples of the various methods used to set up accounts for the Plan.

Types of Account Structures

Contract Administrator Owns Account

The Contracted Administrator has the account and requires the Plan Sponsor to transfer funds whether Wire Transfer, ACH or check directly to them. If a check is written the Contracted Administrator will require the check to be made payable to them. This method may in fact be deemed to allow the Contracted Administrator ownership of the funds. Many plans will have this method of fund transfer for the plan. *This structure is **not** recommended*. The following is an illustration of this Account Structure where the Plan Sponsor receives the billing from the Contracted Administrator and sends the funds to the Contracted Administrator for the Plan. Request a copy of the account ownership with the Bank for validation.

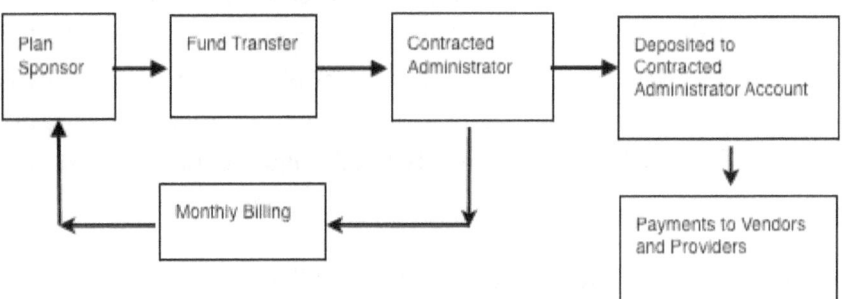

If this method is used, check to see if the Contracted Administrator is providing check registers for the payments to vendor of the plan, Medical Providers, Prescription Benefits (PBM). If the Plan Sponsor is not receiving the check registers, then request the check registers from the Contracted Administrator. The check registers compared to the deposits and the initial forensic evaluation of the Stoploss, Funding,

Vendor Payments, Payments to Providers, Prescription Benefit Payments, Stoploss Reimbursements, and PBM Rebates. This comparison should match the balance of funds.

Note: This method is normally used in the account structure when there are mark ups in the vendor agreements held by the Contracted Administrator and commingling of funds with other plans under the Contracted Administrator. This type of arrangement will normally not have the checks issued for payment in a consecutive order. This account structure will help mask the mark ups in the vendor payments which are considered non disclosed compensation vs disclosed compensation.

A request of copies of check payments to vendors and payments to providers to the plan is warranted. These copies will show the accounts from where the payments originated. There may be more than one account involved.

Example: The Contracted Administrator receives the funds from the Plan Sponsor. The contracted Administrator may have the Vendor Payments placed in their account and pay the net cost to the vendors to the plan while the Contracted Administrator retains the difference and places the funds used to pay providers in another account. If this becomes fact then a request to the vendors of the plan is warranted, requesting copies of billings to the plan and validation payments received. This will validate non disclosed compensation or disclosed compensation.

Request Monthly Bank Statements for the Plan from the Contracted Administrator.

Contract Administrator Sets Up FBO Account

The Contracted Administrator sets up an FBO account in the name of the Plan Sponsor. The Contracted Administrator requires the Plan Sponsor to transfer funds whether Wire Transfer, ACH or check directly to the Account. If a check is written, then the check is made payable to the FBO Account.

This method will allow the Contracted Administrator full access to the funds. Many plans will have this method of account structure for the plan. This structure is better than the funds being owned by the Contracted Administrator. The following is an illustration of this Account Structure where the Plan Sponsor receives the billing from the Contracted Administrator and sends the funds to the FBO Account for the Plan. Request a copy of the account ownership with the Bank for validation.

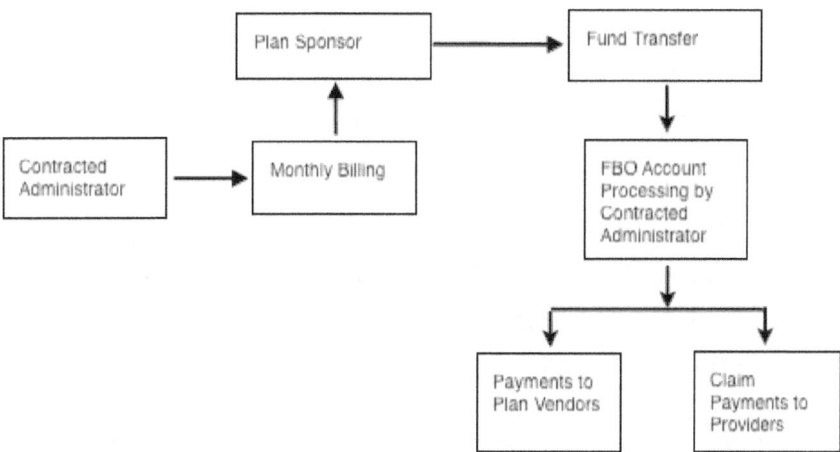

If this method is used, check to see if the Contracted Administrator is providing check registers for the payments to vendors of the plan, Medical Providers, Prescription Benefits (PBM) to the Plan Sponsor. If the Plan Sponsor is not receiving the check registers, then request the check registers from the Contracted Administrator. The check registers compared to the deposits and the initial forensic evaluation of the Stoploss, Funding, Vendor Payments, Payments to Providers, Prescription Benefit Payments, Stoploss Reimbursements, and PBM Rebates. This comparison should match the balance of funds in the FBO Account.

With this account structure, the checks written should be in consecutive order. The potential remains with the payments to the vendors in markups. If the Contracted Administrator is writing one check for fees payable to them for the vendors to the plan and then states they are writing the checks to the vendors, the potential exists for non-disclosed compensation.

This vendor payment structure will help mask the markups in the vendor payments which are considered non disclosed compensation vs disclosed compensation.

A request of copies of check payments to vendors is warranted. These copies will show the accounts from which the payments made are originated from and will validate the non disclosed or disclosed compensation to the Contracted Administrator. There may be more than one account involved.

Example: The Contracted Administrator process the payments from the funds in the FBO Account. The contracted Administrator may write a check to themselves for the Vendor Payments and deposit this transaction in their account and then pay the net cost to the vendors of the plan. *The Contracted Administrator retains the difference.* If this becomes fact, then a request to the vendors of the plan is warranted requesting copies of billings to the plan and validation payments received. This will validate non disclosed compensation or disclosed compensation.

Request monthly bank statements for the Plan from the Contracted Administrator.

Plan Sponsor Establishes Account and Contracted Administrator establishes FBO Account.

The Plan Sponsor establishes the account for the Plan at the bank of their choice. The Plan Sponsor Account requires all vendor payments to be made from the Plan Sponsor Account. The Contracted Administrator sets up an FBO account in the name of the Plan Sponsor for processing of claims. The Contracted Administrator requires the Plan Sponsor to transfer funds whether Wire Transfer, ACH or check directly to the FBO Account. If a check is written, then the check is made payable to the FBO Account.

This method will allow the Contracted Administrator full access to the funds for processing the claim payments for the Plan. Many plans will have this method of account structure for the plan. This structure is better than the funds being owned by the Contracted Administrator. The following is an illustration of this Account Structure where the Plan Sponsor receives the billing from the Contracted Administrator and deposits funds in the Plan Sponsor Account and transfers the funds to the FBO Account for the claim payments for the Plan. Request a copy of the account ownership with the Bank for validation on both accounts.

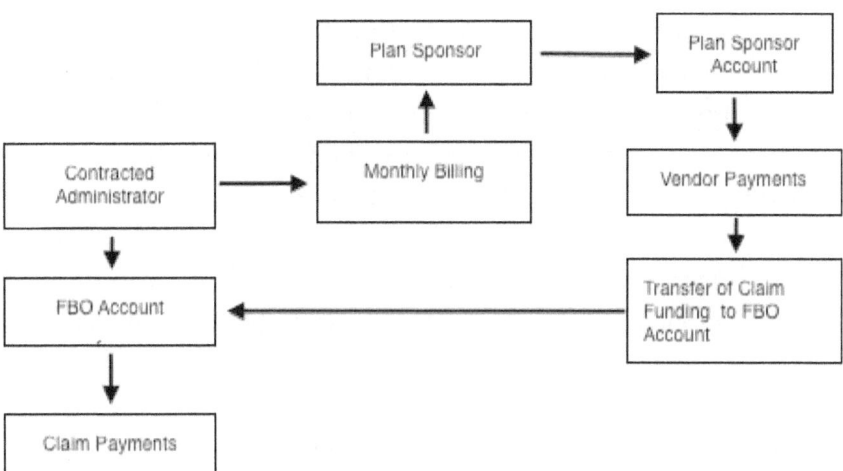

If this method is used, the Contracted Administrator should be providing check registers for the payments to vendors of the plan. The FBO Account should provide check registers on claims paid to Medical Providers, Prescription Benefits (PBM) to the Plan Sponsor. If the Plan

Sponsor is not receiving the check registers, then request the check registers from the Contracted Administrator.

The check registers from each account are used to compare the deposits and the initial forensic evaluation of the Stoploss, Funding, Vendor Payments, Payments to Providers, Prescription Benefit Payments, Stoploss Reimbursements, and PBM Rebates. This comparison should match the balance of funds in the FBO Account.

This vendor payment structure will help reduce the markups in the vendor payments which are considered non disclosed compensation vs disclosed compensation.

Example: The Plan Sponsor deposits the funds based on the billing from the Contracted Administrator. The Contracted Administrator should provide a check register for the vendor payments and the funds to be transferred to the FBO Account. The Contracted Administrator receives a check for the administrative fees and each vendor receives a check for their fees / Stoploss Premiums. This structure reduces the likelihood of markups. However, the vendors to the plan may be providing a compensation check to the Contracted Administrator once they receive the payment. If this becomes fact, then a request to the vendors of the plan is warranted requesting copies of billings to the plan and validation payments received and compensation paid to the Contracted Administrator. This will validate non disclosed compensation or disclosed compensation.

Request monthly bank statements for the Plan from the Plan Sponsor and Contracted Administrator for the respective accounts.

Plan Sponsor Establishes Accounts

The Plan Sponsor establishes the account for the plan at the bank of their choice. The Plan Sponsor Account requires all vendor payments and Providers Payments to be made from the Plan Sponsor Account.

The Plan Sponsor establishes a Deposit Account with two $0 Daily Deposit Accounts (DDA) accounts, One DDA account will be for vendor payments and the second will be for claim payments. The Contracted Administrator sets up the accounts in their system for processing of vendor payments and claims. The Plan Sponsor requires all check registers to be submitted and approved prior to the Contracted Administrators release of checks for each of the respective accounts.

The Contracted Administrator only has the ability to process on the $0 DDA accounts and has no access to the deposit account. This account structure is the best basis for the Plan Sponsor as they control all aspects of the account.

This method will allow the Contracted Administrator to process the vendor payments and claim payments for the Plan without access to the funds of the accounts. This structure is the best for the plan accounts. The following is an illustration of this Account Structure where the Plan Sponsor receives the billing from the Contracted Administrator and deposits funds in the Plan Sponsor Deposit Account. The payments to the vendors and providers for claims are processed on the respective DDA accounts. When checks are presented for payment an automatic transfer takes place to fund the $0 DDA account. The Plan Sponsor remains in control of all funds. Request a copy of the account which will show the Plan Sponsors ownership with the Bank for validation on the accounts.

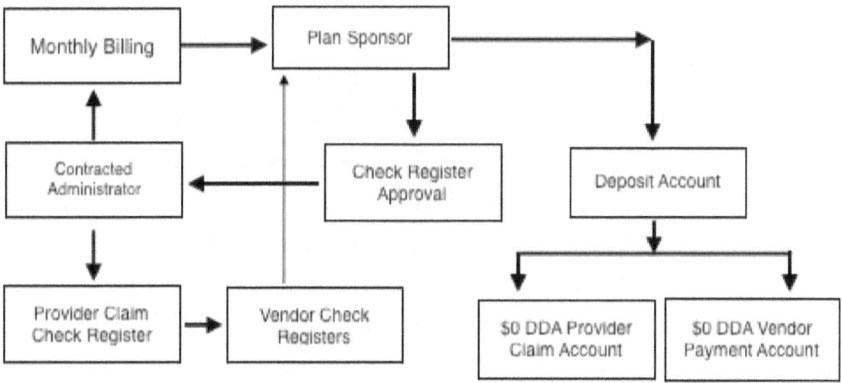

The proper method for this structure is the Contracted Administrator, ASO (Insurance Company) or TPA (Third Party Administrator) based, on an expense (vendor) or claim (provider) check run to submit the detailed check register to the Plan Sponsor for approval and release of the checks. This structure will give the appropriate accounting for all claims and expenses the plan incurs. The Contracted Administrator should have the capabilities to transmit the information on the check register for the expense or claim in a spreadsheet. This is normally standard and available from any Claims system in today's administrative environment. The import of this information to an accounting program such as a QuickBooks or another system will allow for the validation and proper accounting of the funds (this will be discussed in the accounting section).

This allows for reports to be generated as well as to view the various parties which are being paid on behalf of the plan as Providers or vendors to the plan. This is only a surface structure as there may be accounting by the various vendors to the plan which may have additional compensation paid to vendors of the plan such as Contracted Administrator, Agents, Brokers, Consultants etc, from the payments to these vendors to the plan.

Example: The Plan Sponsor / Fiduciary in the establishment of the account is to structure a Deposit Account for all expenses to be deposited from the billing invoice. Set up a zero balance DDA Account as the payment account which has the Contracted Administrator as a signature. Based on the check register presented by the Contracted Administrator, an amount equal to the approved check register would be transferred to the DDA account for release and payment of claims / expenses for the plan as presented. Some Plan Sponsors set up 2 DDA Accounts - one for the fixed expenses and one for the claim expenses. The Contracted Administrator would have these accounts set up appropriately in their system for payment of expenses or claims from the respective account. Thus, the Plan Sponsor / Fiduciary funds have now been protected and in the event there is a termination of the Contracted Administrator. The Plan Sponsor can shut down the account and establish new account(s) for DDA with the new Contracted Administrator. This keeps a separation of the processes done by each entity. Of course the deposit account would not need to be changed as this is an internal account and the Contracted Administrator has no access to it.

Request monthly bank statements for the Plan from the Plan Sponsor for the respective accounts.

Another acceptable method is when the plan sponsor establishes their own account at the bank of their choice without the DDA accounts. ***This type of structure provids simplicity to the accounting and is usually preferred by the plan sponsor for the health plan account.*** The following diagram shows the process for the health plan account.

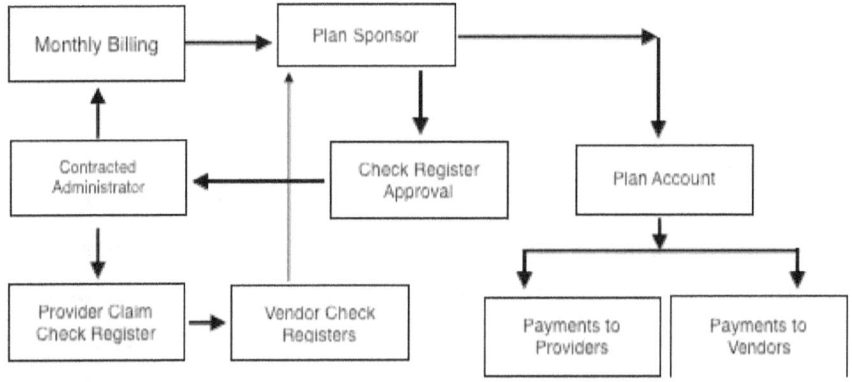

Accounting

The accounting process for validation needs to be set up properly. Many practices use QuickBooks Pro and has been very easy. Use the software most comfortable and confident for you. In setting up the accounting, the following will need to be established depending on the structure of the type of Account structures previously discussed. Set up the Chart of Accounts. The chart of accounts listed below are from a case that was investigated. The chart of accounts can be expanded to encompass each area (category for the plan). For example in professional fees, if an Employee Assitance Program (EAP) is part of the Plan, then the Professional Fees would be expanded to include the EAP Fees.

Bank - Accounts established by Account Structure. An example of the process used in the Account Structure: Plan Sponsor Establishes Account and Contracted Administrator establishes FBO Account. Lets assume the Plan Sponsor Account is with US Bank and the FBO Account established by the Contracted Administrator is with Wells Fargo Bank.

Bank Accounts

Any Bank USA (Plan Sponsor Account)

Account	Type
Health Plan Account	Bank
Medical Claim Refund	Income
Claim Refunds	Income
Audit Recovery	Income
Subrogation Recovery	Income
Prescription Claim Refund (Rebates)	Income
Stoploss Reimbursements	Income
Specific Stoploss	Income
Aggregate Stoploss	Income
Bank Service Charges	Expense
Insurance Expense	Expense
Stoploss Premium	Expense
Specific Stoploss	Expense
Aggregate Stoploss	Expense
Aggregate Accommodation	Expense
Medical Claims	Expense

Prescription Claims	**Expense**
Professional Fees	**Expense**
Consultant Fees	**Expense**
COBRA Fees	**Expense**
Medical Administration Fees	**Expense**
PBM Fees	**Expense**
PPO Fees	**Expense**
Special Program Fees	**Expense**
UR/PreCert/CM/DM/NL Fees	**Expense**

The Chart of Accounts above will normally accommodate the various income and expenses to the Plan. This is only a guide and the chart of accounts can be adjusted with additions or deletions to meet the structure of the plan.

With the Chart of Accounts established, the entry of the check registers and deposits are done. This can be a tedious exercise but must be done for validation. If the Contracted Administrator can provide the check registers for each of the accounts in a spreadsheet, this may create the ability to import the registers to the bank account.

The check register for the Plan Sponsor Account in this case will include the fees paid to the various vendors to the Plan under Professional Fees. From the Parties / Vendors to the Plan form completed initially will allow for placement of the vendor to the appropriate Expense Accounts. Set each of the parties of the plan up as vendors and check off in the set up of the vendors 1099 eligible. This will become important when reviewing the 5500 Form, Schedules A and C for the plan. This will also place a validation in a comparison to the 1099's produced by the Contracted Administrator. This information will also provide validation to the Forensic Dissection of Fees, Premiums and compensation for the Plan.

The check register for the claims will include medical claims and prescription claims. This will become important when a comparison is done for validation on the claim expenses to the plan with application to Aggregate Stoploss as well as the Specific Stoploss claims.

In the forensic basis of the accounting, records should be requested from the various vendors to the plan for compensation, rebates, and other fees. being paid to other vendors of the plan for compensation. This information is then compared to the disclosure of compensation declared by various vendors to the plan. In many instances, compensation will be found which is not disclosed to the Plan Sponsor/Trustees and can be considered as potential fraud. Remember, the Plan falls under ERISA for Self Funded Plans and should be considered as fraud for the instance of non disclosure to the Plan Sponsor / Fiduciary of the Plan. Thus, this structure for analytics is comparing various documentation to the actual variance of the documentation to compensation, fees and commissions.

Not only does this apply to the vendors of the Plan but also an internal evaluation of the funds for proper depositing vs actual deposits for the plan. During investigations, findings from this structure have shown deficits in this analysis and may require an additional deposit or a refund of over deposits as to the differences found to provide an accurate basis for the funding of the plan.

A secondary validation for internal structures for the fixed costs allows for the validation of the 1099 payments to vendors which is reflected on the 5500 Form under Schedule A for supporting vendor payments as well as Schedule C for Administrative cost. This validation is also used when a vendor to the plan wants to audit their fees to the plan which is also based on a month to month eligible census for the proper calculation and payment to the respective vendor.

A summary report for this structure can be accomplished by the proper compilation of this information.

In addition to the above which is an overall view of what is occurring with the plan a more in-depth structure is required for the forensic view of the various vendors associated with the plan which will provide information for compensation and fees. This forensic view will uncover the disclosed compensation as well as the undisclosed compensation which may be paid by the vendor to another representative to the plan such as a TPA, ASO, Agent, Broker, consultant or others. This dissection will provide the objective information which will show additional cost that can reduce or eliminate the undisclosed fees / commission being paid and allow for a better construction of the vendors by providing full transparency and allowing for the best possible outcomes for the plan.

From the findings there may be an indication of fraud. This is normally exposed from the findings when one of the parties to the plan intentionally deceives the Plan Sponsor / Fiduciary when the receipt of money or other benefits are not rightly theirs based on Agreements.

There are red flags which arise that may indicate the potential of fraud. These are based on the facts and circumstances from the initial findings that will require further investigation based on the nature of the objective information found. The red flags are merely an indicator that further investigation into the circumstances is required due to the severity of findings. This may require bringing in a Special Investigation Unit from the respective Department of Insurance or FBI and the facts given to this unit from the initial findings.

The forensic analysis by utilization of the accounting processcan expose the potential for fraud. The types of fraud which may be exposed are Hard Fraud, Soft Fraud or Opportunistic Fraud or all of these Fraud Structures. These type of fraud structures may be internal or external to the plan. To understand the meanings of these types of fraud an explanation is noted:

Hard Fraud

In a health benefit plan fraud can be committed from within the Plan Sponsor, Administrator whether a TPA or ASO or others associated with the plan. An example of this type of fraud can be caused by the contact person internally with the Plan Sponsor or Administrator by receipt of kick backs from vendors.

Soft Fraud

In a health benefit plan fraud can occur from within the Plan Sponsor, Administrator a TPA or ASO, an Agent, Broker or Consultant or another vendor to the plan. This is usually due to the padding or addition to fees which are non disclosed. This can also occur in the underwriting process for non disclosure of information. This can be due to only showing the participating employee census vs the full eligible census, non disclosure of requested high claimants for underwriting of the plan. In addition, some fraud has been seen from Agents, Brokers and Consultants changing the DOB in the census to get a better rate. The soft fraud is also know as an opportunistic fraud. This opportunistic fraud is usually related to economics. As an example, an Administrator, Agent, Broker or Consultant may not disclose pertinent information to an underwriter just to get the business or compensation for placing the plan. This is done by providing false information to obtain lower rates by the manipulation or false information to an underwriter to increase the acceptance of the application for coverage. This type of fraud is more widespread than hard fraud. This type of soft fraud can be very costly to a plan if a claim for Stoploss is made. This can result in the revocation of the Stoploss coverage and place an extreme financial burden on the plan, plan sponsor and fiduciaries as they will have to cover the expenses without coverage of Stoploss.

Fraud in whatever form found ultimately creates higher cost to the plan which is paid for by the Plan Sponsor and its participants to the plan.

This type of fraud is one of the most costly types of fraud in the United States and effects all parties involved.

These are only a few examples of fraud. Fraud can also occur with the falsification of claims by a provider. These and other types of fraud create more investigation requirements and may involve the FBI.

Bank Account Analytics

Setting the Chart of Accounts properly and input of data provide an objective analysis of the finances for the self funded health plan. In this exercise the proper input of the financial information on the self funded health plan is critical when providing analysis and the objective facts report for the self funded health plan. The properly structured input of data as well as the extraction of this data properly placed into the structured reports for each of the vendor architecture as well as aggregate and specific Stoploss will provide the actual loss ratios based on claims, refunds, rebates, medical and prescription.

Note: Requesting the copies of the bank statements and reconciliation gives an objective base for the validation of the transactions for the plan.

We will view the chart of accounts in order to show the proper documentation for the self funded plan.

Health Plan Deposits

This account records the actual deposits the plan made for each period of contribution. The plan year may be on a calendar (January 1 to December 31) or fiscal year (July 1 to June 30).

Date	Number			Payment	Deposit	Balance
01/15/2016		Any Plan Sponsor USA		X	$21,600.00	$21,600.00
	DEP	Health Plan Deposit	January 2016			

This transaction provides the date of deposit, the amount of the deposit, the category in the chart of accounts and the time period. The x or check mark will show this has been reconciled with the bank statement. The extraction of the deposit data will show each period and will be able to be compared to the actual requirement based on the participating census and corresponding allocations for the plan. This information can be placed in the report showing the contribution compared to the actual contribution required.

The following is extracted from the analytical report showing the required deposit vs the actual deposit. The * denotes contributions made in addition to the actual required self funded health plan contribution and should be noted in the report as listed below. This report will not show the PBM Rebates or other income to the plan as this is contained in a separate report. The report below only shows the required deposit to the plan based on cost structured, census count by category vs actual deposit / contribution made. This is important as it applies to the requirement by the Stoploss carrier and plan sponsor in calculation of the contractual agreement for validation of contributions required vs actual contributions made by the plan. This primarily affects the calculation for specific and aggregate reimbursements if there is a claim to the Stoploss carrier for reimbursements to the plan. The example below shows the Plan Sponsor owes the plan $18,700.21 to make it whole.

Required vs Actual Deposits

PLAN SPONSOR (PS) 2015 Exposure vs Deposits - Health Plan			
Month	Exposure (Required)	Actual Deposit	Difference (+) PS Owes Plan (-) Plan Owes PS
*July	$23,639.63	$18,385.00	$5,254.63
August	$23,639.63	$21,995.00	$1,644.63
September	$24,136.19	$22,055.00	$2,081.19

October	$24,136.19	$22,025.00	$2,111.19
*November	$24,136.19	$21,600.00	$2,536.19
December	$24,136.19	$21,600.00	$2,536.19
January	$24,136.19	$21,600.00	$2,536.19
February	$0.00		$0.00
March	$0.00		$0.00
April	$0.00		$0.00
May	$0.00		$0.00
June	$0.00		$0.00
Totals	$167,960.21	$149,260.00	$18,700.21

Setup Fee - $1,500 made in addition to deposit *July 2015

PPACA Transitional Reinsurance Fee - November 2015 - $2,508.

PICORI Fee - Additional TBD

The information for the calculation of the required contributions utilizes an initial report for census calculation by participating category and the detailed vendor contributions required.

Census by participation category

Month	EE	ES	EC	Family	Total
July	43	0	3	1	47
August	43	0	3	1	47
September	43	0	2	2	47
October	43	0	2	2	47
November	43	0	2	2	47
December	43	0	2	2	47
January	43	0	2	2	47
February	0	0	0	0	0
March	0	0	0	0	0
April	0	0	0	0	0
May	0	0	0	0	0

June	0	0	0	0	0
Total	301	0	16	12	329
Mo. Avg.	43	0	2	1.71	47

Vendor Premium and Fees

Category	EE	ES	EC	Family
Stoploss Spec	$110.09	$214.85	$190.66	$320.45
Stoploss Agg	$10.50	$10.50	$10.50	$10.50
Aggregate Accom.	$1.50	$1.50	$1.50	$1.50
Aggregate Funding	$298.43	$594.47	$526.13	$892.90
Plan Admin w/ COBRA	$20.75	$20.75	$20.75	$20.75
UR Precert	$3.50	$3.50	$3.50	$3.50
PPO	$4.90	$4.90	$4.90	$4.90
Broker / Consultant	$16.50	$16.50	$16.50	$16.50
Total	$466.17	$866.97	$774.44	$1,271.00

This extracted table brings in the calculation from the above tables on census and vendor fees / premiums.

Month	Stoploss	Plan Admin	UR Precert	PPO	Broker / Consultant	Monthly Agg	Total Exposure
July	$6,190.30	$975.25	$164.50	$230.30	$775.50	$15,303.78	$23,639.63
August	$6,190.30	$975.25	$164.50	$230.30	$775.50	$15,303.78	$23,639.63
September	$6,320.09	$975.25	$164.50	$230.30	$775.50	$15,670.55	$24,136.19
October	$6,320.09	$975.25	$164.50	$230.30	$775.50	$15,670.55	$24,136.19
November	$6,320.09	$975.25	$164.50	$230.30	$775.50	$15,670.55	$24,136.19
December	$6,320.09	$975.25	$164.50	$230.30	$775.50	$15,670.55	$24,136.19
January	$6,320.09	$975.25	$164.50	$230.30	$775.50	$15,670.55	$24,136.19
February	$0.00	$0.00	$0.00	$0.00	$0.00	$0.00	$0.00
March	$0.00	$0.00	$0.00	$0.00	$0.00	$0.00	$0.00
April	$0.00	$0.00	$0.00	$0.00	$0.00	$0.00	$0.00
May	$0.00	$0.00	$0.00	$0.00	$0.00	$0.00	$0.00
June	$0.00	$0.00	$0.00	$0.00	$0.00	$0.00	$0.00
Total	$43,981.05	$6,826.75	$1,151.50	$1,612.10	$5,428.50	$108,960.31	$167,960.21
Mo. Avg.	$6,283.01	$975.25	$164.50	$230.30	$775.50	$15,565.76	$23,994.32

The information in this chart is utilized in the actual calculation and payments to the various vendors per their contracts with the self funded health plan. This chart may be expanded for Stoploss by providing actual categories for Specific Premium, Aggregate Premium and Aggregate Accommodation. Additionally, the Plan Administration can be expanded by using the categories of Plan Administration and Cobra Administration. The chart above aggregates these costs to the plan.

The following is a extracted report from accounting showing the contributions made by the plan sponsor for the self funded plan.

Type	Date	Name	Memo	Split	Amount	Balance
Deposit	07/22/15	Plan Sponsor	July 2015 Binder Premium	Any Bank USA	6,190.3	6,190.3
Deposit	07/22/15	Plan Sponsor	TPA Admin Set Up Fees	Any Bank USA	1,500	7,690.3
Deposit	08/05/15	Plan Sponsor	July 2015	Any Bank USA	12,194.7	19,885
Deposit	09/03/15	Plan Sponsor	August 2015	Any Bank USA	18,170	38,055
Deposit	09/24/15	Plan Sponsor	September 2015	Any Bank USA	22,055	60,110
Deposit	09/24/15	Plan Sponsor	August 2015 Additional	Any Bank USA	3,825	63,935
Deposit	10/07/15	Plan Sponsor	October 2015	Any Bank USA	22,025	85,960
Deposit	11/06/15	Plan Sponsor	November 2015	Any Bank USA	21,600	107,560
Deposit	11/30/15	Plan Sponsor	December 2015	Any Bank USA	21,600	129,160
Deposit	01/11/16	Plan Sponsor	January 2016	Any Bank USA	21,600	150,760
Total Health Plan Deposits					150,760	150,760
Total Income					150,760	150,760

The accounting provides an overview of the plan and the transactional structure. This information will be utilized in the investigation for fraud in investigation of the transactions by vendor. This will be analyzed in the chapter on FRAUD.

This information shows a total contribution of $150.760.00 vs a total exposure of $167,960.27. The difference is $17,200.27. The set up fee was $1,500 which is not a required contribution and should be considered separate under the plan for contractual contribution purposes. Thus, the contribution for the self funded health plan is $150,760.00 - $1,500 = $149,260. Therefore, the difference from total eposure of $167,960.27 - actual health plan contribution of $149,260 = $18,700.27. As the forensic consultant the analytic calculation ***must*** be accurate for the actual plan contribution. The $18,700.27 is a contractual requirement to be deposited to the plan.

Medical Claim Refund

The medical claim refund can have several areas from which they can be derived. These are return of over payments, subrogation, and recovery of claim payments in excess from audit of claims and claim errors.

When making the memo, it is important to note the participant which the medical claim refund is applied to. This allows the calculation correction in the specific and aggregate Stoploss exposure as a reduction. A notation of the date of claim, claim number, check number, provider and reason for the refund should be recorded.

Date	Number			Payment	Deposit	Balance
01/15/2016		Any Plan provider USA		X	$560.00	$560.00
	DEP	Medical Claim Refund	John Doe, 9/22/2015, Claim 124879A original check 13283, over pmt.			

Claim Refund is a refund of a paid claim which may have been paid twice by the contracted administrator to a provider. The provider returns the overpayment of the claim to the plan.

Claim Recovery is the paying on an inaccurate claim, claim error and then trying to recover the money.

Subrogation is the substitution of one person for another, or of one person into the place of another with respect to rights, claims, or securities. It is most commonly found in the context of insurance, whereby an insurer, having paid a claim to its insured (e.g., automobile collision, workers' compensation, health insurance, etc.) steps into the shoes of its insured and enforces a claim against a third-party tortfeasor, (a person or entity who commits a tort), responsible for causing the loss, in the name of the insured. (https://en.wikipedia.org/wiki/Subrogation)

Claim refunds, recovery and subrogation are applied back to the plan for reduction of plan financial exposure and reduction of loss ratios for the plan and Stoploss ratios for specific and aggregate calculations.

Prescription Claim Refund (Rebates)

Rebates are provided by the manufactures of prescriptions. These are normally based on name brand and formulary drugs. There is a significant dollar range in these rebates. There are several methods for rebates such as full pass through, guaranteed rebates by the PBM (Prescription Benefit Manager) as well as various other methods for providing rebates. These rebates are part of the plan and should be paid to the plan. Rebates are applied to reduce the exposure of the Stoploss for the plan. Rebates when provided in the proper basis provides the name of the participant and the rebates associated with this individual so they can be applied to both the specific and aggregate Stoploss in the reduction of exposure. This creates better loss ratios for the plan and reduces exposure for the Stoploss on both the specific.

Note: In many instances, the plan sponsor may sign an agreement that provides the rebates to be paid to the PBM, ASO (Administrative Services Only) normally provided by an insurance company, TPA (Third Party Administrator) or Agent / Broker or Consultant. At times these rebates may be shared by all above leaving out the plan sponsor. It is important to read the agreements to make sure the rebates are provided back to the plan as the plan who own the rebates. Plan sponsors will sign agreements not knowing what they have signed and forfeit the rebates to one or all of the parties above.

Date	Number			Payment	Deposit	Balance
01/15/2016		Prescription Benefit Management		x	$1,190.00	$1,190.00
	DEP	Prescription Claim Refund (Rebate)	3rd qtr - July to September 2015			

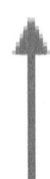

Rebate reports should include the individual names and listed in the splits for each individual to have the proper allocation against the prescription claims, thus creating a reduction in claims by applying a reduced exposure for the Stoploss both on a specific and aggregate level.

Rebates, depending of the agreement may be applied as a point of service (POS), or provided as a check to the plan sponsor when correctly contracted

Additionally, rebates may be contracted as a full pass through to the plan sponsor, or contracted as guaranteed rebates. Contracted rebates in the contract / agreement provide a risk basis to the PBM and plan sponsor. If the guaranteed rebates are less than the actual rebates then the PBM keeps the difference and the plan sponsor receives the guaranteed rebate. If the guaranteed rebates are more than the actual rebates, the PBM loses and the plan sponsor keeps the guaranteed rebates.

The timing on the various types of rebates mentioned are:

POS provides the calculated rebates on each eligible prescription as the transaction occurs. The POS rebates are normally less than the contracted rebates and actual rebates.

The *contracted rebates* are normally provided at the end of the following quarter and paid by a check. These rebates may be more or less than the actual rebates

The *actual rebates* are normally paid anywhere from 9 to 12 months after the eligible prescriptions have been paid and is paid by a check. These rebates may be more or less than the contracted rebates.

Refunds are normally applied to the current billing and provide a credit on the amount of the prescription billing. The prescription billing is handled in the same process as the rebates for allocation to the proper individual providing a reduction in Stoploss on a specific and aggregate basis. These are normally entered in the Prescription claims chart of accounts based on the billing. Splits will be used in the application of these refunds when entering the amounts for each individual in the accounting.

Stoploss Reimbursements are applied when the Stoploss exposure limits are exceeded by the plan. These are broken down into two categories - Specific Stoploss and Aggregate Stoploss.

Date	Number			Payment	Deposit	Balance
01/15/2016		Stop Loss Carrier		x	$8,206.00	$8,206.00
	DEP	Stop Loss Reimbursement - Specific Stop Loss	Participant Name			

Stoploss on the Specific reimbursement may be on several individuals and should be listed in the splits with the sub category of Specific Stoploss Reimbursement. This allows for the proper allocation to the individual(s) which exceeded the plan exposure limits on the plan. These reimbursements are used to reduce the Stoploss exposure on the Aggregate Stoploss with regard to the plan.

SUMMARY TOTALS JANUARY 2015 TO DECEMBER 31, 2015 SPECIFIC STOP LOSS ANALYSIS					
Name	Claims Pd	Spec Stop Loss	Over Spec	Amount Reimb.	Amount Due Plan
John Doe	$44,571.69	$40,000.00	$4,571.69	0	$4,571.69
John Smith	$38,269.33	$25,000.00	$13,269.33	$10,744.45	$2,524.88
Totals	$82,841.02		$17,841.02	$10,744.45	$7,096.57

The above is an extraction from the reporting on specific Stoploss claims on individuals under the plan. The report shows the amounts of the specific deductible and the reimbursements received as well as reimbursements due. The example above shows the Stoploss limits by individual, one for $40,000 which is considered a laser to the plan on the specific Stoploss individual above the Stoploss contracted limit in this example of $25,000.

Note: It is important to read the Stoploss agreement to know if the plan has any contengencies for individual(s) with a laser. Additionally, it is also important to read the basis on which the specific Stoploss reimbursements will be paid out. Some Stoploss contracts will state that once the specific Stoploss is exceeded by $2,000 this must occur before the reimbursements will be paid. Others will have $0 exceeded before the specific Stoploss reimbursemrnt is paid to the plan.

Stoploss on the Aggregate reimbursement is based on the exposure to the plan exceeding the Aggregate Attachment Point on the plan. Aggregate Stoploss Attachment point has a basis of the cash from $0 up to the specific Stoploss deductible and then aggregated for the Attachment point limit in reduction of exposure to the plan for risk management. The following report is extracted from the reports for the plan.

Plan Sponsor Aggregate Reimbursements Received 2013 Plan Year Stop Loss Carrier

Stop Loss Aggregate Accommodation Received 2013

Month	Monthly Aggregate	Med/Rx Net	Date Received	Check #	Agg Reimbursement	Summary Balance
January	$14,083.80	$1,398.75			$ 0.00	$12,685.05
February	$14,083.80	$29,053.85			$ 0.00	-$14,970.05
March	$14,083.80	$23,931.54			$ 0.00	-$9,847.74
April	$14,083.80	$68,244.22	4/25/13	3613	$ 11,989.34	-$42,171.08
May	$14,553.51	-$15,269.66	5/28/13	3645	$ 20,673.62	$50,496.79
June	$14,553.51	$17,170.00			$ 0.00	-$2,616.49
July	$14,553.51	$23,783.98			$ 0.00	-$9,230.47
August	$14,553.51	-$5,003.45	8/13/13	3570	$ 5,872.21	$25,429.17
September	$13,144.38	$13,190.86			$ 0.00	-$46.48
October	$12,674.67	$16,146.68			$ 0.00	-$3,472.01
November	$12,674.67	$53,935.98			$ 0.00	-$41,261.31
December	$13,144.38	-$42,053.51			$ 0.00	$55,197.89
Totals	$166,187.34	$184,529.24			$ 38,535.17	$20,193.27

This example shows the monthly aggregate, the net Medical and Prescription claims. The net Medical and Rx Claims take into account specific Stoploss reimbursement paid and Prescription rebates. The Aggregate Reimbursements have two ways of being applied - If the plan sponsor has chosen aggregate accommodation the reimbursements are paid during the plan year to provide risk management for the cash flow of the plan. Utilizing the aggregate accommodation provision basically provides a loan to the plan and any amounts in excess of the actual aggregate exposure at the end of the plan year must be paid back to the Stoploss carrier. In the example report above, the aggregate has a summary balance of $20,193.27 and this money must be paid back to the Stoploss carrier to reduce the summary balance to $0.

Aggregate Stoploss reimbursements not utilizing the aggregate accommodation are paid at the end of the plan year. The plan sponsor must fund the amounts in excess during the plan year and file for reimbursements at the end of the plan year.

Date	Number			Payment	Deposit	Balance
05/28/2013		Stop Loss Carrier		x	$20,673.62	$20,673.62
	DEP	Stop Loss Reimbursement - Aggregate Stop Loss Reimbursement	Plan Year Applied to			

The entry into the accounting should state the plan year applied in the memo section. This will allow the proper allocation in the plan year to which the aggregate reimbursement should be applied.

Note: It is important to read the Stoploss Agreement for the aggregate Stoploss. Additionally, it is also important to read the basis on which the aggregate Stoploss reimbursements will be paid out. Some Stoploss contracts will state the aggregate Stoploss must be exceeded by $5,000 before reimbursements will be paid. There is an application in the aggregate Stoploss agreement using a minimum attachment point and/or the actual attachment point. The minimum attachment point is applied in the aggregate contract based on the initial census by category and has an actual allocation of the census by category of participants during the first month of the plan year. The secondary method is the actual census by category by month for allocation of the attachment point. If the census is less than the minimum attachment point in the aggregate Stoploss agreement, the minimum attachment point will apply. This also goes forward in the calculation if the census were to drop during the year. The caluclation for aggregate reimbursement will use the minimum attachment point by contract or the actual attachment point and apply whichever is the greater amount.

Insurance Expenses are broken down in the chart of accounts for Stoploss premium with three subsections Specific Stoploss, Aggregate Stoploss and Aggregate Accomodation. Many times these premiums are combined for accounting purposes; however, the proper basis is to break them out by subsection in the chart of accounts. Entry for the payment of the Stoploss Premium is normally provided in a vendor check register from the Contracted Administrator and is then entered into the accounting for the plan.

Date	Number			Payment	Deposit	Balance
12/22/2015	12512	Stop Loss Carrier		$6320.09 X		$6,320.09
		Stop Loss Premium	December 2015			

The total for the Stoploss is entered into the payment section. The category Stoploss premium is selected and the date is entered for the month to which the Stoploss payment is applied. The premiums are then entered into the Splits section of the accounting to provide the proper accounting for the Stoploss premium. The Splits entry will be shown as follow:

Account	Amount	Memo	Customer Job
Specific Stop Loss	$5756.09	December 2015	
Aggregate Stop Loss	$493.50	December 2015	
Aggregate Accommodation	$70.50	December 2015	

By entry of the splits in accounting a more accurate record of the Stoploss Premium Expense exists and provides for the period which the premiums are allocated and paid. This becomes important when a Stoploss carrier wants proof the premiums were paid and allocated for validation of any Stoploss reimbursements.

The following extract from the accounting report shows the transactional base for the payment of the Stoploss Premiums.

Stop Loss Premium

Type	Date	Num	Name	Memo	Split	Amount	Balance
Check	07/22/15	2	Stop Loss Carrier	July 2015	Any Bank USA	6,190.30	6,190.30
Check	09/03/15	1000	Stop Loss Carrier	August 2015	Any Bank USA	6,449.88	12,640.18
Check	09/22/15	1043	Stop Loss Carrier	September 2015	Any Bank USA	6,320.09	18,960.27
Check	10/13/15	1066	Stop Loss Carrier	October 2015	Any Bank USA	6,320.09	25,280.36
Check	11/12/15	1112	Stop Loss Carrier	November 2015	Any Bank USA	6,320.09	31,600.45
Check	12/22/15	1177	Stop Loss Carrier	December 2015	Any Bank USA	6,320.09	37,920.54
Total Stop Loss Premium						37,920.54	37,920.54
Total Insurance Expense						37,920.54	37,920.54

A detailed report can be printed from the accounting system showing each of the transactions in detail providing the actual allocation to each category in the Stoploss chart of accounts.

Medical Claims entry is based on the check register received from the Contracted Administrator. The following is a sample of what a claims check register should include at a minimum. This check register is an extract from an actual claim register with the names changed the participants, and is used only as an example to show the actual entry in the accounting system.

Claim Check Register

CHKNO	GRPNO	CLMNO	CHKDT	AMT	PAYEE	FIRSTNAME	LASTNAME	FROMDT
1202	5200	8000416	1/8/16	$17.22	SIGNATURE MEDICAL GROUP	DAISY	JONES	12/30/15
1203	5200	8000412	1/8/16	$24.00	DESLOGE VISION CENTER	ROBIN	BIRD	12/14/15
1204	5200	8000415	1/8/16	$30.36	QUALITY HEALTH CARE	JENNIFER	RICHY	12/29/15
1205	5200	8000414	1/8/16	$34.00	REITER CHIROPRACTIC	JOHN	SMITH	12/29/15
1205	5200	8000414	1/8/16	$34.00	REITER CHIROPRACTIC	ROBIN	BIRD	7/8/15
1206	5200	8000417	1/8/16	$78.50	ST. ANTHONY'S KENNERLY FAMILY MEDICINE	CARDINAL	RED	12/14/15
1207	5200	8000411	1/8/16	$111.73	METRO OBGYN	JANE	DOE	12/29/15
1208	5200	8000413	1/8/16	$16.66	QUEST DIAGNOSTIC	JANE	DOE	12/16/15
1208	5200	8000413	1/8/16	$14.17	QUEST DIAGNOSTIC	MARY	SMITH	12/19/15
1208	5200	8000413	1/8/16	$83.33	QUEST DIAGNOSTIC	JANE	DOE	12/8/15
1208	5200	8000413	1/8/16	$51.31	QUEST DIAGNOSTIC	JANE	DOE	12/8/15
1208	5200	8000413	1/8/16	$7.19	QUEST DIAGNOSTIC	JANE	DOE	12/8/15
1209	5200	8000418	1/8/16	$2,232.99	MAXOR PLUS	EXPENSE	EMPLOYEE	12/21/15

The above check register is the minimum that should be received as paid claims for the self funded health plan. In viewing this check register, there are several claims which have the same check number to the provider. These are combined into one check using the split category to allocate to each of the plan participants for that check number.

NOTE: It is important to view the from date (FROMDT) which is the date the claim was incured. A comparison to the Specific Stoploss and Aggregate Stoploss is required to see if the date of service is within the parameters of the Stoploss Agreements. If it is within the dates of the Stoploss contract the individual is listed in the memo field without the FROMDT. If the transaction is out of the parameters of the Stoploss contracts, then the date should be listed after the participants name in the memo field. This will provide additional information needed when a detailed report is done and sorted by participant in the accounting detailed reports for allocation to the specific and aggregate claims.

A normal entry for claims with in the Stoploss contract provisions is:

Date	Number			Payment	Deposit	Balance
01/08/2016	1202	SIGNATURE MEDICAL GROUP		$17.22 X		$17.22
		Medical Claims	Daisy Jones			

Claims which are listed with the same check numbers should be entered on the following basis using the splits for entry.

Date	Number			Payment	Deposit	Balance
01/08/2016	1208	QUEST DIAGNOSTIC		$172.66 X		$172.66
		Medical Claims	Daisy Jones			

The following shows the splits for check number 1208.

Account	Amount	Memo	Customer Job
Medical Claims	$16.66	Jane Doe	
Medical Claims	$14.17	Mary Smith	
Medical Claims	$83.33	Jane Doe	
Medical Claims	$51.31	Jane Doe	
Medical Claims	$7.19	Jane Doe	

If all dates are with in the contract period, then Jane Doe's claims in this split can be combined showing only two entries in the splits for check 1208.

Account	Amount	Memo	Customer Job
Medical Claims	$158.49	Jane Doe	
Medical Claims	$14.17	Mary Smith	

As an example, should one of the claims be out of date with the Stoploss contract, either specific or aggregate, then the detail should be used with the date of claim after the name of the participant in the memo field. For example, if the date on Jane Doe's claim on the $83.33 was incurred on June 2, 2015 would be considered out of contract for specific and/or aggregate Stoploss purposes based on a Stoploss contract which is a July 1, 2015 to June 2016, and would be shown as listed below for the split:

Medical Plan Forensics

Account	Amount	Memo	Customer Job
Medical Claims	$16.66	Jane Doe	
Medical Claims	$14.17	Mary Smith	
Medical Claims	$83.33	Jane Doe 6/2/2015	
Medical Claims	$51.31	Jane Doe	
Medical Claims	$7.19	Jane Doe	

This becomes important when providing the findings which will be discussed in the Reporting Chapter in this book.

Prescription Claims are done on the same basis as the medical claims. In the previous listed claims check register it listed MaxorPlus which is the PBM (Prescription Benefit Manager) for the Self funded health plan. The extraction from the claims register shows:

Claim Check Register

CHKNO	GRPNO	CLMNO	CHKDT	AMT	PAYEE	FIRSTNAME	LASTNAME	FROMDT
1209	5200	8000418	1/8/16	$2,232.99	PBM PLUS	EXPENSE	EMPLOYEE	12/21/15

This register is normally followed by a detailed report which shows the plan participants to which the claims are applied.

Prescription Claim Detail Register

Name	Rx Date	Rx No	Pharmacy	Qty	Days Supply	Copay	Plan Paid	Claim Fee	Amt Due
MARY SMITH	12/23/15	6082671*	CLARK'S RX	0	0	$ 0.00	$ 0.00	$ 0.00	$ 0.00
MARY SMITH	12/23/15	6085441	CLARK'S RX	30	30	$ 10.00	$ 5.16	$ 0.00	$ 5.16
MARY SMITH	12/23/15	6082671	CLARK'S RX	30	30	$ 10.00	$ 1.60	$ 0.00	$ 1.60
CARDINAL RED	12/16/15	2485930	WALGREENS	-30	0	$(10.00)	$ (8.73)	$ 0.00	$ (8.73)
JOHN DOE	12/23/15	6081096	SCHNUCKS	30	30	$ 35.00	$2,198.92	$ 0.00	$2,198.92
JOHN DOE	12/23/15	6081097	SCHNUCKS	60	30	$ 10.00	$ 31.53	$ 0.00	$ 31.53
JANE DOE	12/20/15	7352170	WALMART	-30	0	$(10.00)	$ (2.30)	$ 0.00	$ (2.30)
JANE DOE	12/21/15	7352170	WALMART	30	30	$ 10.00	$ 2.30	$ 0.00	$ 2.30
ROBIN BIRD	12/27/15	1736421*	WALGREENS	0	0	$ 0.00	$ 0.00	$ 0.00	$ 0.00
ROBIN BIRD	12/27/15	1736421	WALGREENS	6	5	$ 10.00	$ 4.51	$ 0.00	$ 4.51

The primary entry is:

Date	Number			Payment	Deposit	Balance
01/08/2016	1209	PBM PLUS		$2232.99	X	$2,232.99
		PRESCRIPTION CLAIMS	January 8, 2016			

The following shows the splits for check number 1209.

Entry of these claims shows what the plan paid for the prescriptions on the split for each participant. If there is $0 no cost for the plan on a participant then that data is not entered. This will include if a prescription was ordered then declined which shows a negative amount for the prescription offsetting the original cost.

Account	Amount	Memo	Customer Job
Prescription Claims	$5.16	MARY SMITH	
Prescription Claims	$1.60	MARY SMITH	
Prescription Claims	-$8.73	CARDINAL RED	
Prescription Claims	$2,198.92	JOHN DOE	
Prescription Claims	$31.53	JOHN DOE	
Prescription Claims	$4.51	ROBIN BIRD	

If all dates are within the contract period, then Mary Smith's claims and John Doe's claims in this split can be combined showing the splits for check 1209.

Account	Amount	Memo	Customer Job
Prescription Claims	$6.76	MARY SMITH	
Prescription Claims	-$8.73	CARDINAL RED	
Prescription Claims	$2,230.45	JOHN DOE	
Prescription Claims	$4.51	ROBIN BIRD	

As an example, should one of the claims be out of date with the Stoploss contract either specific or aggregate then the detail should be used with the date of claim after the name of the participant in the memo field.

For example if the date on John Doe's claim on the $31.53 was incurred on June 2, 2015 which would be considered out of contract for specific and or aggregate Stoploss purposes based on a Stoploss contract which is a July 1, 2015 to June 2016 would be shown as listed below for the split:

Account	Amount	Memo	Customer Job
Prescription Claims	$6.76	MARY SMITH	
Prescription Claims	-$8.73	CARDINAL RED	
Prescription Claims	$2,198.92	JOHN DOE	
Prescription Claims	$31.53	JOHN DOE 6/2/2015	
Prescription Claims	$4.51	ROBIN BIRD	

This becomes important when reporting.

Professional Fees are the vendors fees to the self funded health plan. These can be expanded in the Chart of Accounts to match the vendors to the plan. These are normally provided in a Vendor Check register for payment by the Contracted Administrator. An example of the Vendor Check Register is listed. Each of the vendors to the plan will be applied to the appropriate Professional Fee subheadings in the chart of accounts.

CHKNO	GRPNO	CLMPRE	CLMNO	CHKDT	AMT	PAYEE	FROMDT
1042	32000	2015	356000480	12/22/15	$7,377.07	STOP LOSS COMPANY	12/1/15
1043	32000	2015	356000483	12/22/15	$114.70	MANAGED CARE COMPANY	12/1/15
1044	32000	2015	356000482	12/22/15	$151.90	AGGREGATOR FOR PPO	12/1/15
1045	32000	2015	356000484	12/22/15	$372.00	CONSULTANT	12/1/15
1046	32000	2015	356000485	12/22/15	$830.00	CONTRACTED ADMINISTRATIVE SERVICES	12/1/15

The accounting entries will be as listed below.

Date	Number			Payment		Deposit	Balance
12/22/15	1042	Stop Loss Company		$7377.07	X		$7,377.07
		Stop Loss Premium	December 2015				

As discussed earlier the Stoploss can be detailed for each of the subchart of accounts under the Stoploss premium.

Date	Number			Payment	Deposit	Balance
12/22/15	1043	Managed Care Company		$114.70 X		$114.70
		Ur/PreCert/CM/DM/NL Fees	December 2015			

Date	Number			Payment	Deposit	Balance
12/22/15	1044	Aggregator for PPO		$151.90 X		$151.90
		PPO Fees	December 2015			

Date	Number			Payment	Deposit	Balance
12/22/15	1045	Consultant		$372.00 X		$372.00
		Consultant Fees	December 2015			

Date	Number			Payment	Deposit	Balance
12/22/15	1046	Contracted Administrator Services		$830.00 X		$830.00
		Medical Administration Fees	December 2015			

Reconciliation of the bank account is necessary for the validation of the transactions. This will provide a consistency from the check registers from the contracted administrator to the transactions processed through the plan sponsors health plan bank account.

Summary

The accounting shows a validating transaction base for the health plan from the check registers provided by the contracted administrator. The process begins with verification of the transactions vs the agreements / contracts per vendor for an objective basis in the analytical comparison.

In addition, the comparative analytics from transactions provide a view of markups or no markups on the disclosed or non-disclosed for vendor architecture vs the actual cost presented by comparative analytics to the actual transactions from the check registers issued by the contracted administrator. Utilization of this information and the process of transactions as applied to each section of the report starts the forensic investigation to all objective based facts. Printing out a detailed profit and loss report provides the information for input to the reports for the investigation.

Medical Plan Detail Report

The Medical Plan Detail Report is a relational data report by which the objective data is entered into the report. The information is pulled from the following reports.

Contracted Administrator - Administrative Service Agreement / Administrative Services Only Agreement

Vendor Agreements

Detailed Billing by month from Contracted Administrator

Stoploss Agreement from Stoploss Carrier

Stoploss Detailed Reimbursement Report from Stoploss carrier

PBM reports including Rebates

Accounting Report

The above reports can and should be expanded as the issue at hand requires. The above reports and agreements are a guide to use as a fundamental base.

The information from each of the above agreements and reports are entered into the Medical Plan Detail Report. This is independent of the reports provided by the Contracted Administrator. The detailed Medical Plan Report will be used in a comparative basis to that of the reports provided by the Contracted Administrator. The comparison and subsequent information from the investigative process will provide a means for comparative analytics to uncover information behind each of the transactions for various levels of investigation of the facts.

The first report is the Detail of Expenses which summarizes the various areas of input to the Medical Detail Plan Report. This report is a relational data report a compilation of facts.

The reports are brokendown into sections to explain the data and the relational basis of the compilation of information.

The first report is the Detail of expenses which captures information from the two input levels utilized:

1. The census count by month which is derived from the Detailed Billing Report.
2. The Plan Cost by category which is derived from the Administrative Service Agreement / Administrative Services Only Agreement, Vendor Agreements, Stoploss Agreements and disclosed compensation agreements (Agents, Brokers and Consultants if provided).

Census Count by Month

The following is an extract from the Census Count by Month.

Month	EE	ES	EC	Family	Total
January	23	1	0	0	24
February	25	1	0	0	26
March	23	1	0	0	24
April	24	0	0	0	24
May	25	0	0	0	25
June	25	0	0	0	25
July	25	0	0	0	25
August	29	0	0	0	29
September	27	0	0	0	27
October	27	0	0	0	27
November	29	0	0	0	29
December	31	0	0	0	31
Total	313	3	0	0	316
Mo. Avg.	26.08	0.25	0	0	26.33

The census count for participation shows each level of participation by month. This is important as these counts will be used in substantiation of the billing to each of the categories in the vendor architecture, minimum aggregate attachment point, and/or actual aggregate attachment point.

Plan Cost Structure

The Plan Cost Structure is extracted from the actual agreements from the Administrative Service Agreement / Administrative Services Only Agreement, Vendor Agreements, Stoploss Agreements and disclosed compensation agreements (Agents, Brokers and Consultants if provided. These cost structures can be expanded to allow for any additional fixed cost basis to the plan. As an example, if the Plan Administration and COBRA processing organizations are different then the category for COBRA Administration can be set up and allocated in the Summarized Detail Report by Month. If the Agent, Broker or Consultant is not based on a fee but a commission, the category can be removed and will be structured as commission in a separate report. The following is the plan cost structure.

Category	EE	ES	EC	Family
Stop Loss Spec	$216.41	$427.95	$364.48	$681.79
Stop Loss Agg	$20.06	$20.06	$20.06	$20.06
Aggregate Accom.	$1.50	$1.50	$1.50	$1.50
Aggregate Funding	$662.47	$1,324.94	$1,126.21	$2,119.91
Plan Admin	$20.00	$20.00	$20.00	$20.00
UR Precert	$3.70	$3.70	$3.70	$3.70
PPO	$4.90	$4.90	$4.90	$4.90
Consultant	$12.00	$12.00	$12.00	$12.00
Total	$941.04	$1,815.05	$1,552.85	$2,863.86

This breaks down the various cost components of the plan to use in the calculation of the summarized detail report. The calculation for each category is multiplied by the census count for the month by category and the result is compiled in each of the summarized detail reports sections. These components of cost can be detailed or summarized. For example the summarization of Stoploss would have the Stoploss Specific, Stoploss Aggregate, Stoploss Aggregate Accommodation added together and multipled by the census count by category, and the summed for the cost of the plan in the month of application. These cost can also be categorized separately if needed due to the issue at hand. The Aggregate Funding also known as the attachment point will always have its own category in the summary of detail report by month. This is due to the information being utilized for calculation in other parts of the Medical Plan Detail Report.

Summarized Monthly Detail Report

This report compiles a summarized monthly report based on the information from the Census Count by Month and the Plan Cost Structures. This report can also be expanded to meet the issue at hand. Detailing all the categories may be a requirement for the issue at hand.

The areas by category are filled in from this report but will **not** include the following categories as these are calculated from other reports as relational. Not included are the Med Paid, Rx Paid, Spec Reimb, Agg Reimb, Rx Rebates as these are compiled in separate reports with the results being shown in the Summarized Monthly Detail Report as a relational basis of data.

The following report is an example of the Summarized Monthly Detail Report based on the information relating to the objective data.

The structure of the report allows the view of the objective data from the census count by month by category and the cost structure by category, compiled into the monthly summarized plan costs.

Plan Sponsor PLAN ANALYSIS JANUARY 1, 2015 THROUGH DECEMBER 31, 2015
Detail Report

Month	Stop Loss	Plan Admin	UR Precert	PPO	Consultant	Monthly Agg	Med Paid	Rx Paid	Spec Reimb	Agg Reimb	RX Rebates	Retention	Total Paid	Total Exposure
January	$5,922.82	$480.00	$88.80	$117.60	$288.00	$16,561.75	$201.34	$2,540.48	$0.00	$0.00	$0.00	$13,729.73	$9,729.24	$20,458.97
February	$6,398.76	$520.00	$96.20	$127.40	$312.00	$17,866.69	$34,706.14	$5,512.00	$0.00	$0.00	$0.00	$-22,331.45	$47,672.50	$25,341.05
March	$5,922.82	$480.00	$88.80	$117.60	$288.00	$16,561.75	$2,896.26	$5,784.06	$0.00	$0.00	$423.00	$8,304.43	$15,154.54	$23,458.97
April	$5,711.28	$480.00	$88.90	$117.60	$288.00	$16,899.28	$1,939.79	$4,943.36	$9,344.90	$0.00	$0.00	$17,941.03	$4,643.92	$22,584.96
May	$5,949.25	$500.00	$92.50	$122.50	$300.00	$16,561.75	$16,334.70	$5,456.52	$0.00	$0.00	$0.00	$-4,228.47	$27,754.47	$23,526.00
June	$5,949.25	$500.00	$92.50	$122.50	$300.00	$16,561.75	$6,358.94	$4,544.60	$0.00	$0.00	$0.00	$5,658.51	$17,867.49	$23,526.00
July	$5,949.25	$500.00	$92.50	$122.50	$300.00	$16,561.75	$20,567.93	$5,356.17	$0.00	$0.00	$0.00	$-9,352.35	$32,878.35	$23,526.00
August	$6,901.13	$580.00	$107.30	$142.10	$348.00	$19,211.63	$3,306.94	$4,235.27	$2,399.95	$0.00	$0.00	$14,066.97	$13,221.19	$27,290.16
September	$6,426.19	$540.00	$99.90	$132.30	$324.00	$17,866.69	$1,329.20	$5,663.58	$0.00	$0.00	$0.00	$10,893.91	$14,514.17	$25,408.08
October	$6,426.19	$540.00	$99.90	$132.30	$324.00	$17,886.69	$2,199.25	$5,510.76	$0.00	$0.00	$0.00	$10,216.68	$15,191.40	$25,408.08
November	$6,901.13	$580.00	$107.30	$142.10	$348.00	$19,211.63	$3,230.70	$3,401.85	$0.00	$0.00	$0.00	$12,609.08	$14,681.08	$27,290.16
December	$7,277.07	$620.00	$114.70	$151.90	$372.00	$20,536.57	$8,412.55	$3,415.27	$5,693.69	$0.00	$0.00	$14,359.44	$14,812.80	$29,172.24
Total	$75,833.14	$6,320.00	$1,199.20	$1,548.40	$3,792.00	$211,327.92	$99,913.64	$56,365.92	$16,396.14	$0.00	$423.00	$71,869.51	$226,121.16	$299,990.67
Mo. Avg.	$6,319.43	$526.67	$97.43	$129.03	$316.00	$17,610.66	$8,326.14	$4,697.16	$1,366.01	$0.00	$35.25	$5,990.13	$19,010.10	$24,999.22

Month	EE	ES	EC	Family	Total
January	23	1	0	0	24
February	25	1	0	0	26
March	23	1	0	0	24
April	24	0	0	0	24
May	25	0	0	0	25
June	25	0	0	0	25
July	25	0	0	0	25
August	29	0	0	0	29
September	27	0	0	0	27
October	27	0	0	0	27
November	29	0	0	0	29
December	31	0	0	0	31
Total	313	3	0	0	316
Mo. Avg.	26.08	0.25	0	0.00	26.33

Category	EE	ES	EC	Family
Stop Loss Spec	$216.41	$427.95	$364.48	$681.79
Stop Loss Agg	$20.06	$20.06	$20.06	$20.06
Aggregate Accom.	$1.50	$1.50	$1.50	$1.50
Aggregate Funding	$662.47	$1,324.94	$1,126.21	$2,119.91
Plan Admin	$20.00	$20.00	$20.00	$20.00
UR Precert	$3.70	$3.70	$3.70	$3.70
PPO	$4.90	$4.90	$4.90	$4.90
Consultant	$12.00	$12.00	$12.00	$12.00
Total	$941.04	$1,815.05	$1,552.85	$2,863.86

2014 Claims	IBNR Medical Not Eligible 2015 Agg	IBNR Rx Not Eligible 2015 Agg	Laser Not Eligible 2015 Agg	Total Not Eligible 2015 Agg
	$22,706.38	$3,710.86	$15,000.00	$41,417.24

Amounts not applied to aggregate but eligible for Specific Stop Loss for 2015 contract

Report Prepared by F. Randall Childers, Jr., CFC - Licensed Employee Benefit Consultant
randall_childers@me.com

As a separate basis from the summary report is a report on IBNR (Incurred But Not Received) and Laser(s). These areas are calculated in a separate relational report and are summarized in the report below Census and Cost. These reports will be discussed and shown as we move to each of the relational categoris in the Medical Plan Detailed Report in its entirety.

From the information compiled in the relational data structure, a Summary Report is produced to show only a year to date summary with corresponding graphs of the break out of the information as a percentage of the totals.

This report summarizes the information in a graph basis and helps to illustrate this data as an overall comparison for the cost and retention of the plan.

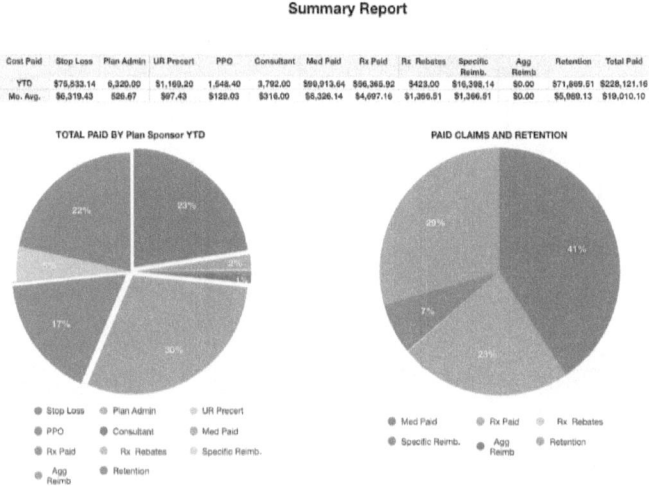

Aggregate Report

The aggregate report compiles the medical and prescription claims by month and applies them against the attachment point less any specific Stoploss reimbursements, prescription rebates, IBNR, and laser exclusions. This provides the loss ratio of the plan. The relation information for each of the above calculations specific Stoploss reimbursements, prescription rebates, IBNR, and laser exclusions are compiled in separate reports but relate the data to the aggregate report. The information with regard to claims are extracted from the accounting report for medical and prescription claims sorted by check run period or by month. The following is an extract of this report.

Aggregate Eligible Claims Report

Plan Sponsor PLAN ANALYSIS JANUARY 1, 2015 THROUGH DECEMBER 31, 2015
Aggregate Stop Loss Report

[Aggregate Stop Loss Report table with monthly claims data for January through December 2015, showing columns for Count, Monthly Aggregate, Monthly Med Claims Inside Aggregate, Monthly Rx Claims Inside Aggregate, Rx Rebates, Monthly Specific Reimb. Amount, Monthly Med Rx Net Claim Subj to Aggregate, YTD Aggregate, Med and Rx YTD Claims Subj to Agg, YTD Summary, and Loss Ratio.]

Report Prepared by F. Randall Childers, Jr., CFC - Licensed Employee Benefit Consultant
randall_childers@me.com

The aggregate eligible claims report will show the claims by check run period and by month. Information is extracted from the IBNR report as well as the Laser Report for application of the net eligible aggregate claims by month and applied to the aggregate report for both medical and prescription claims.

The claims for medical and prescription are extracted from the accounting by separate report for each and sorted by date which will provide the claims paid for each of the check run periods. This information is entered into the Aggregate Eligible Claims Report.

> **Aggregate eligible claims = total claims - IBNR Claims - (incurred prior to contract period) - Laser(s) (amounts over contracted Stoploss).**
>
> **To get total expenses for period add Total MM and Total Rx. This will provide total claims paid by plan for each month. This total should match the paid claims in the accounting system.**
>
> **To get total expenses for YTD add Total MM and Total Rx. This will provide total claims paid by plan YTD. This total should match the paid claims in the accounting system.**

The information from this report is extracted for the Aggregate Report to show the actual eligible aggregate claims for medical and prescription **after** reductions for IBNR and LASERS.

The paid claims for the medical and prescription should match the accounting information for medical and prescription claims **before** any reductions for IBNR, LASER. or Specific Stoploss Reimbursements.

The following is an extract of Aggregate Eligible Claims report.

Plan Sponsor PLAN ANALYSIS JANUARY 1, 2015 THROUGH DECEMBER 31, 2015
Aggregate Eligible Claims

Plan Sponsor Aggregate Eligible Claims Report 2015

Month	MM 1	MM 2	MM3	MM4	Total MM	Less IBNR	Less Laser	Eligible Total MM
January	$138.03	$2,820.06	$9,066.48		$12,027.17	$11,755.60	$0.00	$291.54
February	$347.24	$492.76	$5,764.81	$33,232.81	$38,807.12	$5,130.98	$0.00	$34,706.14
March	$11.98	$747.81	$164.56	$2,235.83	$3,160.16	$253.82	$0.00	$2,866.36
April	$937.11	$2,439.62	$370.49	$558.57	$4,205.79	$2,845.00	$0.00	$1,360.79
May	$2,958.03	$10,833.86	$2,562.39	$653.75	$16,879.51	$1,444.81	$0.00	$15,334.70
June	$562.19	$363.76	$3,318.01	$2,207.90	$6,451.66	$93.02	$0.00	$6,358.64
July	$187.03	$3,547.69	$3,863.76	$13,039.76	$20,674.93	$117.00	$0.00	$20,557.93
August	$1,832.25	$136.75	$526.43	$1,066.81	$3,306.94	$0.00	$0.00	$3,306.94
September	$514.35	$100.00	$4,140.99	$281.88	$5,037.22	$431.46	$3,276.56	$1,329.20
October	$2,474.60	$542.07	$2,137.78	$980.24	$5,384.60	$230.00	$2,990.41	$2,169.25
November	$729.67	$214.29	$3,400.50	$0.00	$4,417.46	$0.00	$1,216.76	$3,200.70
December	$6,199.36	$1,319.10	$4,402.83	$4,464.09	$16,137.38	$213.00	$7,511.27	$8,412.55
Totals YTD	[illegible]	[illegible]	[illegible]	[illegible]	[illegible]	[illegible]	[illegible]	[illegible]

Month	RX 1	Rx 2	Rx 3	Rx 4	Total Rx	Less IBNR	Eligible Total Rx
January	$3,710.86	$2,540.48	$0.00	$0.00	$6,251.34	$3,710.86	$2,540.48
February	$2,289.50	$3,222.50	$0.00	$0.00	$5,512.00	$0.00	$5,512.00
March	$2,483.22	$3,300.84	$0.00	$0.00	$5,784.06	$0.00	$5,784.06
April	$2,639.04	$2,304.32	$0.00	$0.00	$4,943.36	$0.00	$4,943.36
May	$2,530.17	$2,925.35	$0.00	$0.00	$5,455.52	$0.00	$5,455.52
June	$1,124.95	$3,419.65	$0.00	$0.00	$4,544.60	$0.00	$4,544.60
July	$1,793.25	$3,592.92	$0.00	$0.00	$5,386.17	$0.00	$5,386.17
August	$2,834.22	$1,391.05	$0.00	$0.00	$4,225.27	$0.00	$4,225.27
September	$2,902.06	$2,791.00	$0.00	$0.00	$5,693.06	$0.00	$5,693.06
October	$1,658.62	$3,852.14	$0.00	$0.00	$5,510.76	$0.00	$5,510.76
November	$767.96	$2,633.90	$0.00	$0.00	$3,401.86	$0.00	$3,401.86
December	$816.50	$2,601.72	$0.00	$0.00	$3,418.27	$0.00	$3,418.27
Totals YTD	[illegible]	[illegible]	$0.00	$0.00	[illegible]	$3,710.86	[illegible]

Aggregate eligible claims = total claims - IBNR Claims - Laser(s) (incurred prior to contract period) - Laser (amounts over contracted stop loss).

To get total expenses for period add Total MM and Total Rx. This will provide total claims paid by plan for each month.

To get total expenses for YTD add Total MM and Total Rx. This will provide total claims paid by plan YTD.

REPORT PREPARED BY: F. RANDALL CHILDERS, JR., CFC, DABFE - LICENSED CONSULTANT - (502) 6743-8739 - RANDALL CHILDERS@ME.COM

3

IBNR Report

The IBNR Report shows claims incurred but not received for the current Stoploss contract for Specific and Aggregate. It is important to know the contract for Stoploss for both specific and aggregate Stoploss contracts. The claims may not be eligible for the aggregate Stoploss contract but may be eligible for the specific Stoploss contract. This occurs when the dates for eligible incurred and paid claims are different.

As an example a Stoploss contract using a calendar year for the specific contract with a run in or run out provision may have those claims incurred in the run in or run out provision eligible due to the dates listed in the Specific ContractIng. The specific contract may be set up for a 15/12 contract which means claims incurred October 1 in the previous year to December 31 of the current year are eligible for the specific Stoploss contract. If the contract is a 12/15 means claims incurred January 1 in the current year to March 31 of the following year are eligible for the specific Stoploss contract. In contrast the Aggregate Stoploss Contract may have no run in or Run out provisions and is based on a 12/12 incurred and paid basis (Incurred January 1 to December 31 and Paid January 1 to December 31) on the current calendar or plan year basis. Thus, claims falling outside these parameters on an incurred basis would not be eligible for the Aggregate Stoploss Contract. *It is very important to know the Stoploss Contract periods for both the Specific Stoploss and Aggregate Stoploss.*

In the accounting entries under the Memo field the name of the individual and the date of the claim on claims incurred outside the contract period are listed. The information is extracted from the medical claims and prescription claims in separate reports. Those claims in the memo field with dates are then extracted and sorted to get those claims considered IBNR and then listed in the IBNR report by check run date. The data from this information is entered into the IBNR Report by check run period and month for calculation and extraction to the Aggregate Report for subtraction to get the eligible aggregate claims.

Additionally, this information is used by participant when entering those claims eligible for the specific Stoploss contract. Claims not eligible for the aggregate Stoploss contract may be eligible for the Specific Stoploss

Contract. *It is very important to know the Stoploss Contract periods for both the Specific Stoploss and Aggregate Stoploss.*

This data is extracted for the IBNR reporting under the detail of expenses listed at the bottom of the report for IBNR Medical and Prescription claims.

An example of the IBNR report is listed below.

Plan Sponsor PLAN ANALYSIS JANUARY 1, 2015 THROUGH DECEMBER 31, 2015
IBNR

Plan Sponsor IBNR Report 2015
Plan Sponsor 2014 Claims in 2015 Not Eligible for 2015 Aggregate

Month	MM 1	MM 2	MM3	MM4	Total MM IBNR	RX 1	Rx 2	Rx3	Rx4	Total Rx IBNR
January	$138.03	$2,822.66	$8,774.94	$0.00	$11,735.63	$3,710.86	$0.00	$0.00	$0.00	$3,710.86
February	$163.60	$299.12	$4,583.26	$85.00	$5,130.98	$0.00	$0.00	$0.00	$0.00	$0.00
March	$11.98	$217.56	$0.00	$34.38	$263.92	$0.00	$0.00	$0.00	$0.00	$0.00
April	$501.38	$2,344.62	$0.00	$0.00	$2,846.00	$0.00	$0.00	$0.00	$0.00	$0.00
May	$27.04	$704.04	$579.68	$334.05	$1,644.81	$0.00	$0.00	$0.00	$0.00	$0.00
June	$0.00	$0.00	$93.02	$0.00	$93.02	$0.00	$0.00	$0.00	$0.00	$0.00
July	$0.00	$0.00	$117.00	$0.00	$117.00	$0.00	$0.00	$0.00	$0.00	$0.00
August	$0.00	$0.00	$0.00	$0.00	$0.00	$0.00	$0.00	$0.00	$0.00	$0.00
September	$0.00	$0.00	$431.46	$0.00	$431.46	$0.00	$0.00	$0.00	$0.00	$0.00
October	$0.00	$0.00	$0.00	$230.00	$230.00	$0.00	$0.00	$0.00	$0.00	$0.00
November	$0.00	$0.00	$0.00	$0.00	$0.00	$0.00	$0.00	$0.00	$0.00	$0.00
December	$213.56	$0.00	$0.00	$0.00	$213.56	$0.00	$0.00	$0.00	$0.00	$0.00
Totals	$1,055.59	$6,388.00	$14,579.36	$683.43	$22,706.38	$3,710.86	$0.00	$0.00	$0.00	$3,710.86

REPORT PREPARED BY: F. RANDALL CHILDERS, JR., CFC, DABFE - LICENSED CONSULTANT - (502) 6743-8739 - RANDALL.CHILDERS@ME.COM

Specific Stoploss Report

The specific Stoploss report shows the participants who exceeded the Stoploss deductible for the plan year. The information for this report is extracted from the accounting for medical and prescriptions and then sorted by participant. This report in its entirety is done with data entered by month for the participants less any IBNR which is outside the dates of the specific Stoploss contract. The information is summarized for a quick view of the amounts above the specific Stoploss deductible for reimbursements.

This report will also bring in the reimbursemnts for Stoploss from the Reimbursement Input report. Remember the information in all the various reports are relational based on the objective data received and inputted into the various reports.

The following report shows a summary but has detail by each participant who exceeded the the Stoploss deductible on a month by month input of the claims. As the data is entered, a report is extracted from the accounting for medical and prescription claims by individual. This report is important as a supplement to specific Stoploss report for the objective data used in the calculation of the specific Stoploss report.

It is very important to know the Stoploss Contract periods for the Specific Stoploss.

\multicolumn{6}{c}{SUMMARY TOTALS JANUARY 2015 TO DECEMBER 31, 2015 SPECIFIC Stoploss ANALYSIS}
Name	Claims Pd	Spec Stoploss	Over Spec	Amount Reimb.	Amount Due Plan
1	$44,571.69	$40,000.00	$4,571.69	$3,775.76	$795.93
2	$38,269.33	$25,000.00	$13,269.33	$12,622.38	$646.95
Totals	$82,841.02		$17,841.02	$16,398.14	$1,442.88

In this summary, participant number 1 has a Laser for $40,000 which is an amount above the contracted Stoploss of $25,000 as shown for participant number 2. The difference is $15,000 for number 1. This $15,000 additional amount is not applied to the aggregate Stoploss and an additional report is needed which is similar to the specific Stoploss report but has a number which is used in calculating the net aggregate claims eligible for the aggregate Stoploss. This report is listed as the LASER Report.

Laser Analysis Report

The laser analysis report provides the proper calculation on the amounts not eligible for the Aggregate Report and is compiled from the data used for claims in the specific report. Thus, the amounts reimbursable from the claims exceeding the specific laser deductible will be the same in the specific deductible report for Specific Stoploss reimbursement. The information from the Laser Analysis Report is relational as the data for the month to month for the amounts exceeding the contracted specific deductible up to the laser specific deductible are calculated and data is extracted to the Aggregate Eligible Claims as a reduction. The information from the Aggregate Eligible Claims (Net) are then incorporated by the relational report to the Aggregate Report. This provides a basis for the Aggregate Stoploss Report also shown as the Aggregate Report. This allows for the proper calculation for loss ratios and will provide the proper data to the Aggregate Stoploss Report. Thus, it is important to read the Stoploss contract for individuals listed with lasers. Some plans may have more than one individual listed with different laser amounts and some plans will not have any lasers.

The following is the extract summary for the laser analysis report.

SUMMARY TOTALS JANUARY 2015 TO DECEMBER 31, 2015 SPECIFIC Stoploss LASER ANALYSIS					
Name	Claims Pd	Spec Stoploss Laser	Over Specific	Stoploss per Agreement	Not Eligible for Aggregate
1	$44,571.69	$40,000.00	$4,571.69	$25,000.00	$15,000.00
	$44,571.69		$4,571.69		$15,000.00

This report shows the amount not eligible for the Aggregate Report. The amount over specific Stoploss limit is the amount to be reimbursed by the specific Stoploss contract to the plan sponsor for risk management of the plan.

Stoploss Specific Reimbursement Report

The specific Stoploss reimbursement report shows the Stoploss reimbursements made to the plan and applied to the individuals which exceeded the specific deductibles or laser. The data is listed in the accounting for Stoploss reimbursements - specific Stoploss.

This information if not provided should be requested from the Stoploss Carrier / MGU (Managing General Underwriter) with copies of the checks and a detail report for each check and claimant report which will show allowed and disallowed claims. If the information is not available from the Stoploss carrier as they have not received any requests for reimbursement, then a problem could exist with the contracted administrator based on not filing the claim(s) with the Stoploss carrier. If this fact is uncovered, the contracted administrator should be questioned as to why this was not done. This could possible be a claim against the Contracted Administrator and their E&O (Errors and Omissions coverage). A note should be included in this report if this is fact.

This report is relational as it extracts the amount of reimbursement(s) due the plan for each of the individuals who have exceeded the specific Stoploss deductible or laser. The information entered into this report will also be provided to the Specific Stoploss Report to show if there are ramining reimbursements due the plan. This information will also show in the Stoploss Reimbursement Report.

Plan Sponsor Specific Reimbursements Received 2015 Plan Year Stoploss Carrier					
Month	Date	Check #	Amount	1	2
Specific Amount			$17,841.02	$4,571.69	$13,269.33
January					
February					
March					
April	04/10/15	1463	$8,344.90		$8,344.90
May					
June					
July					
August	08/24/15	1489	$2,399.55		$2,399.55

September						
October						
November						
December						
Jan 1, 2015	01/29/16	1526	$1,877.93		$1,877.93	
Feb 1, 2015	01/29/16	1535	$3,775.76	$3,775.76		
Total Reimbursed			$16,398.14	$3,775.76	$12,622.38	
Difference to Plan Reimbursable			$1,442.88	$795.93	$646.95	

The report indicates the date the check was written, check number and total amount. Then allocation is made on the participants who exceeded the specific deductible or laser and indicates the amount still due the plan and remaining amounts on the claims filed on each participant. The reimbursed amounts are relational to the aggregate report showing the specific Stoploss reimbursements which reduce the aggregate Stoploss calculation.

Aggregate Reimbursement Report

This report brings in the actual attachment point for the plan with the medical and prescription net claims. The summary balance shows the basis for potential aggregate Stoploss reimbursements for the plan by indication of a negative number. It is important to view the total under the summary balance for a total negative number. The medical and RX will be offset by specific Stoploss reimbursements to be applied to the aggregate report as well as any PBM (Pharmacy Benefit Manger) rebates received by the plan. If there is an aggregate reimbursement to be received by the plan due to a negative number, the check and the amount of reimbursement will be entered into this report. This reimbursement should show the summary balance as $0 once received. If after receipt of the aggregate reimbursement the summary balance shows as a positive number, the positive amount is to be returned to the Stoploss carrier with a report attached showing the calculation and subsequent return of funds to the Stoploss carrier. Due to the relational basis of this data, the monthly aggregate is relational to the monthly aggregate calculated from the Detail of Expenses report under the heading monthly aggregate.

Plan Sponsor Aggregate Reimbursements Received 2015 Plan Year Stop Loss Carrier			Plan Sponsor Aggregate Accommodation Received 2015			
Month	Monthly Aggregate	Med/Rx Net	Date Received	Check #	Agg Reimbursement	Summary Balance
January	$16,561.75	$2,832.02			$ 0.00	$13,729.73
February	$17,886.69	$40,218.14			$ 0.00	-$22,331.45
March	$16,561.75	$8,257.32			$ 0.00	$8,304.43
April	$15,899.28	-$2,041.75			$ 0.00	$17,941.03
May	$16,561.75	$20,790.22			$ 0.00	-$4,228.47
June	$16,561.75	$10,903.24			$ 0.00	$5,658.51
July	$16,561.75	$25,914.10			$ 0.00	-$9,352.35
August	$19,211.63	$5,142.66			$ 0.00	$14,068.97
September	$17,886.69	$6,992.78			$ 0.00	$10,893.91
October	$17,886.69	$7,670.01			$ 0.00	$10,216.68
November	$19,211.63	$6,602.55			$ 0.00	$12,609.08
December	$20,536.57	$6,177.13			$ 0.00	$14,359.44
Totals	$211,327.93	$139,458.42			$ 0.00	$71,869.51

From the information above, the comparison to the aggregate minimum attachment point is necessary in application of the data to see if the minimum aggregate attachment point is greater than the actual attachment point. If the minimum attachment point is greater than the actual aggregate point and a negative balance is shown, then this amount will be used to determine the aggregate Stoploss reimbursement to the plan and or the amount to be returned to the Stoploss carrier if after the reimbursement is received and the summary balance amount is a positive balance.

Aggregate Minimum Attachment Report

It is important to read the Stoploss agreement for the aggregate coverage to determine the minimum attachment point for the plan. Many times a total amount is indicated in the Stoploss agreement for the minimum aggregate attachment point which is divided by 12 to obtain the monthly minimum aggregate attachment point. In the language within the Stoploss for the aggregate attachment point, a calculation may be indicated for application to the first month census and then calculated against the attachment point factors and then multiplied by 12 to obtain the minimum aggregate attachment point for the plan. This caluclation is then divided by 12 to obtain the monthly minimum aggregate attachment point for application. The following is the aggregate minimum attachment point.

A comparison for the actual attachment point and minimum attachment point is necessary. If the actual attachment point based on the calculation of the monthly participation multipled by the attachment point factors is greater than the minimum attachment point factors then the greater amount is used for the calculation and vise versa for the comparison of the attachment point factors.

With these two reports, the aggregate attachment point for the plan is $211,372.03 is greater than the minimum attachment point of $206,690.64. Thus, the actual aggregate attachment point is used for the calculation in determining if there is an aggregate Stoploss reimbursement is warranted.

Stop Loss Aggregate Contracted Minimum Attachment Point

Month	Minimum Attachment Point	Med/Rx Net	Summary Balance	Aggregating Balance
January	$17,224.22	$2,832.02	$14,392.20	$14,392.20
February	$17,224.22	$40,218.14	-$22,993.92	-$8,601.72
March	$17,224.22	$8,257.32	$8,966.90	$365.18
April	$17,224.22	-$2,041.75	$19,265.97	$19,631.15
May	$17,224.22	$20,790.22	-$3,566.00	$16,065.15
June	$17,224.22	$10,903.24	$6,320.98	$22,386.13
July	$17,224.22	$25,914.10	-$8,689.88	$13,696.25
August	$17,224.22	$5,142.66	$12,081.56	$25,777.81
September	$17,224.22	$6,992.78	$10,231.44	$36,009.25
October	$17,224.22	$7,670.01	$9,554.21	$45,563.46
November	$17,224.22	$6,602.55	$10,621.67	$56,185.13
December	$17,224.22	$6,177.13	$11,047.09	$67,232.22
Totals	$206,690.64	$139,458.42	$67,232.22	

Deposit Report

If there is an aggregate Stoploss reimbursement to be applied to the plan, the MGU (Managing General Underwriter) for the Stoploss carrier will require a report to validate the Plan Sponsor has met their obligation for funding the actual aggregate attachment point or minimum aggregate attachment point on the basis of which one is greater. The information is extracted from the accounting report for deposits to the plan by the plan sponsor. A calculation is then made to validate the plan sponsor has deposited the proper amount for the plan for the aggregate funding of the plan. This validation is necessary before any aggregate Stoploss reimbursements are made by the Stoploss carrier. The following will show the comparison from the actual deposits made vs. the required deposits for the aggregate attachment point calculation. Remember the basis for this is the objective data for the plan.

The following is an extract from the accounting on the actual deposits made reduced by the fixed cost of the plan for vendor fees and Stoploss premiums and fees. This will provide the actual deposit for the aggregate attachment point made by the plan sponsor.

							03/16/16
Type	Date	Num	Name	Memo	Split	Amount	Balance
Deposit	01/02/15	DEP	Plan Sponsor	January 2015 StopLoss Binder	Any Bank	6,161	6,161
Deposit	01/09/15	DEP	Plan Sponsor	January 2015 Funding	Any Bank	17,704.15	23,865.15
Deposit	02/06/15	DEP	Plan Sponsor	February 2015	Any Bank	25,283.08	49,148.23
Deposit	03/09/15	DEP	Plan Sponsor	March 2015	Any Bank	23,626.97	72,775.2
Deposit	03/26/15	DEP	Plan Sponsor	April 2015	Any Bank	20,000	92,775.2
Deposit	03/26/15	DEP	Plan Sponsor	April 2015	Any Bank	2,752.96	95,528.16

Deposit	05/11/15	DEP	Plan Sponsor	May 2015	Any Bank	23,700	119,228.16
Deposit	06/01/15	DEP	Plan Sponsor	June 2015	Any Bank	23,700	142,928.16
Deposit	07/06/15	DEP	Plan Sponsor	July 2015	Any Bank	23,700	166,628.16
Deposit	08/14/15	DEP	Plan Sponsor	August 2015	Any Bank	27,482.16	194,110.32
Deposit	09/14/15	DEP	Plan Sponsor	September 2015	Any Bank	26,535.12	220,645.44
Deposit	10/15/15	DEP	Plan Sponsor	October 2015	Any Bank	25,588.08	246,233.52
Deposit	11/13/15	DEP	Plan Sponsor	November 2015	Any Bank	28,588.16	274,821.68
Deposit	12/15/15	DEP	Plan Sponsor	December 2015	Any Bank	29,382.24	304,203.92
						304,203.92	304,203.92

From the accounting report for deposits, the monthly actual aggregate is extracted as shown in the following report.

Plan Sponsor 2015 Required vs Actual Deposits for Aggregate - Health Plan

Month	Aggregate Funding Exposure (Required)	Actual Deposit	Less fees, Stoploss Premiums,	FSA Fees	ACA Fees	Actual Deposit for funding aggregate exposure	Difference (+) Plan Sponsor Owes Plan (-) Plan Owes Plan Sponsor
January	$16,561.75	$23,865.15	$6,897.22	$168.00		$16,799.93	-$238.18
February	$17,886.69	$25,283.08	$7,454.36	$180.00		$17,648.72	$237.97
March	$16,561.75	$23,626.97	$6,897.22	$168.00		$16,561.75	$0.00
April	$15,899.28	$22,752.96	$6,685.68	$168.00		$15,899.28	$0.00
May	$16,561.75	$23,700.00	$6,964.25	$174.00		$16,561.75	$0.00
June	$16,561.75	$23,700.00	$6,964.25	$174.00		$16,561.75	$0.00
July	$16,561.75	$23,700.00	$6,964.25	$174.00		$16,561.75	$0.00
August	$19,211.63	$27,482.16	$8,078.53	$192.00		$19,211.63	$0.00
September	$17,886.69	$26,535.12	$7,521.39	$186.00	$941.04	$17,886.69	$0.00
October	$17,886.69	$25,588.08	$7,521.39	$180.00		$17,886.69	$0.00
November	$19,211.63	$28,588.16	$8,078.53	$198.00	$1,100.00	$19,211.63	$0.00
December	$20,536.57	$29,382.24	$8,635.67	$210.00		$20,536.57	$0.00
Totals	$211,327.93	$304,203.92	$88,662.74	$2172.00	$2,041.04	$211,328.14	-$0.21

This comparison shows the plan sponsor made the required deposits for the aggregate attachment point. The expenses paid are validated against the accounting. Thus, a validation from the calculation for proper deposits made to the aggregate exist on the objective facts.

PBM Rebate Report

The PBM Rebate shows the rebates received for the plan. It is important to read the agreements for Administration and the PBM Agreement for rebates. Many Contract Administrators and PBM's will retain these rebates per the agreements. Rebates depending on how the PBM proceeses them may take up to a year to receive payment. Thus, if rebates are to be paid to the plan, it is important to get copies of the rebate checks and for the period for which they apply. This will provide data tracking on any rebates received by the plan. Rebates are used in reducing the aggregate for the plan when and if received. Thus, rebates will lower the exposure on the aggregate and will provide an improvement in the loss ratio for the aggregate calculation. The rebates also play a role in determining the amount of aggregate reimbursement due to the reduction of the claims cost by application. This information is also based on a relational basis for the reports for Aggregate and the Detail of Expenses report. The following shows the PBM Rebate Report for the plan. The rebate report will show the date the rebate was received with the check number, the amount and which quarter it was applied.

Plan Sponsor Rebates Received for RX 2015 PY				
	Date Received	Check #	Amount	Qtr Applied
January				
February				
March	12/16/15	51184	$423.00	1st qtr 2015
April				
May				
June				
July				
August				
September				
October				
November				
December				
Total			$423.00	

Fraud in Self Funded Medical Plans

From the findings there may be an indication of fraud. This is normally exposed from the findings when one of the parties to the plan intentionally deceives the Plan Sponsor / Fiduciary when the receipt of money or other benefits are not rightly theirs.

A good definition of Fraud as stated by WebCE, Inc. and International Risk Management Institute, Inc. (IRMI) in their CE on Insurance Fraud published in 2016:

"Fraud is any deliberate act of deceit, falsehood, or other dishonest undertaking perpetrated against or by and insurance company or its agents for the purpose of unwarranted financial gain."

This definition can be adapted to self funded plans by adding vendors to the plan after the insurance company. This is due to the fact that anyone who seeks unwarranted financial gain through various means is committing fraud.

Using the methods and tools in this book will help to detect fraud... The accounting tools, forensic decision mapping, review of agreements, reports, documents and the disclosure of affidavits on compensation paid to or received by a vendor to the plan or provider.

There are red flags which arise that may indicate the potential of fraud. These are based on the facts and circumstances from the initial findings that will require further investigation based on the nature of the objective information found. The red flags are merely an indicator that further investigation into the circumstances and severity of the findings may be needed. This may require bringing in a Special Investigation Unit from the respective Department of Insurance and issuing the factual report based on initial findings.

The forensic analysis by utilization of the accounting can expose the potential for fraud. The types of fraud which may be exposed are Hard Fraud, Soft Fraud or Opportunistic Fraud or contribution of these fraud structures. These types of fraud structures may be internal or external to the plan. To understand the meanings of these types of fraud an explanation is noted:

Hard Fraud

In a health benefit plan hard fraud may be committed from within the Plan Sponsor, or Administrator whether a TPA or ASO or others associated with the plan. An example of this type of fraud can be caused by the contact person internally with the Plan Sponsor or Administrator by receipt of kick backs from vendors.

Soft Fraud

In a health benefit plan, soft fraud may occur from within the Plan Sponsor or Administrator whether a TPA or ASO, an Agent, Broker or Consultant or another vendor to the plan. This is usually due to the padding or additional fees which are non-disclosed. This can also occur in the underwriting process for non disclosure of information. This can be due to only showing the participating employee census vs the full eligible census, non disclosure of requested high claimants for underwriting of the plan. In addition, some fraud has been seen by Agents, Brokers and Consultants changing the DOB in the census to get a better rate. The soft fraud is also know as an opportunistic fraud. This opportunistic fraud is usually related to economics. As an example an Administrator, Agent, Broker or Consultant may not disclose pertinent information to an underwriter just to get the business or compensation for placing the plan. This is done by providing false information to obtain lower rates by the manipulation or false information to an underwriter to increase the acceptance of the application for coverage. This type of fraud is more widespread than hard fraud. This type of soft fraud can be very costly to a plan if a claim for Stoploss is made. This can result in the revocation of the Stoploss coverage and place an extreme financial burden on the plan, plan sponsor and fiduciaries as they will have to cover the expenses without coverage of Stoploss.

Fraud in whatever form f ultimately creates higher cost in the plan which is paid for by the Plan Sponsor and/or its participants to the plan. This type of fraud is one of the most costly types of fraud in the United States and effects all parties involved.

These are only a few examples of fraud. Fraud can also occur with the falsification of claims by a provider. This and other types of fraud create more investigation requirements and may involve the FBI.

Documents and Agreements

The documents and agreements to a plan are very important to analyze. When looking at the financial basis of the plan for payments to vendors, compensation for agents, brokers and consultants there is a need to review the documents and agreements for disclosed compensation. There have been many instances where, contracted administrators whether or not a TPA or an ASO have markup agreements with the vendors to the plan when they are bundled. Additionally, agents, brokers and consultants have also had the TPA or ASO add additional compensation which is not disclosed to the Fiduciaries of the plan. Additionally, the TPA or ASO may have added in their fees due to the agent, broker and consultant and do not want the plan sponsor to know what their compensation is for the plan in terms of their commissions or fees. Experience has shown the opportunistic representatives who practice this method do not think they will get caught. By direct analyzation of the agreements and affidavits as the vendors to the plan, full objective disclosure of these types of activities are found and exposed.

The following is an example: A PBM is a vendor which typically is in the middle of financial activity regarding the prescriptions cost, administrative cost sharing with TPA's, ASO's, agents, brokers and consultants. Experience has shown the addition of $.25 to $1.00 per prescription for compensation has been madewithout disclosure to the plan sponsor. Additionally, the rebates (refunds from manufacturers) have been distributed via TPA's, ASO's, agents, brokers and consultants which become compensation to these vendors to the plan. Normally, this type of compensation is not fully disclosed. Rebates are the property of the plan (Plan Sponsor) when self-funded and should be paid to the plan at 100% of the rebates. PBM's try to state they will pay 100% of the eligible rebates (which sounds good on the surface) but the real basis is what is determined as "eligible". The word eligible is normally not defined and is up to the TPA or ASO if the PBM vendor is bundled under the purview of the TPA or ASO to determine how much if any to share with the Plan Sponsor. Additionally, agents, broker or consultants may bring a PBM to the Plan and state they are independent, but in reality, there may be an agreement for compensation on a per prescription basis, and the agent, broker or consultant are keeping the rebates.

The above show the opportunistic structure for the deliberate act of deceit, falsehood, or other dishonest undertaking perpetrated against the Plan or Plan Sponsor for the purpose of unwarranted financial gain.

The following is the Forensic Decision Mapping regarding a PBM and Rebates. Remember, based on information received the algorithm may be expanded.

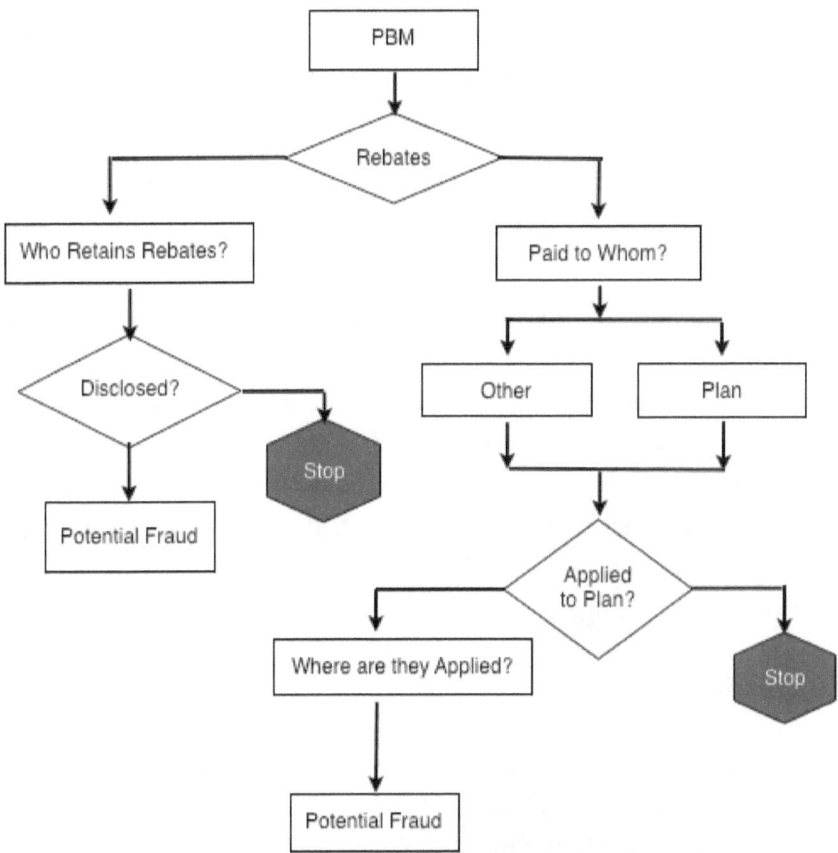

Those who operate with integrity and proper regulatory ethics will disclose this information and will work for the benefit of their client and its participants. The following will discuss additional areas of potential fraud.

Vendor Fraud

When a Plan Sponsor receives their quote from the agent, broker or consultant there is usually no discussion as to compensation built into the Stoploss Insurance or Vendor Fees. Most Plan Sponsors accept the quote based on price alone as long as the benefit plan is similar to their current plan. Since this is a Self-Funded Plan, the Plan Sponsor has a fiduciary responsibility to the plan members to do what is in their best interest. The following is a scenario of an actual case. The names have been changed but the facts are shown as they were discovered.

Case Scenario

This case involves the Plan Sponsor, TPA (Owner), Stoploss Carrier and Agents to the Plan. This case shows the intricacy and deception which can take place due to the Greed Factor. The volume of information and the discovery of the different parties involvement were quite significant. As in the previous chapters, the use of gathering the information and techniques for analysis all were utilized in this case. Each vendor and their information agreements, reports, memos [internal and external] as well as correspondence was used and applied to the Forensic Decision Mapping. Extracts from these mappings will be included in this scenario with the names changed.

Origination

Agent 1 approached the Marketing Director of the TPA to get a quote for a self funded plan with Stoploss for their client who, at this time, was fully insured. The Marketing Director provided a list of information needed to get the quotes from the various underwriters. Agent 1 provided the information and the Marketing Director proceeded to compile the information to be sent to various underwriters for RFQ (Request for Quote).

The owner of the TPA directed the Marketing Director to send the RFQ out to a new underwriter/Stoploss carrier that the TPA had just done an agreement with and had a previous relationship. The marketing director did a search for this new underwriter / Stoploss carrier on AM Best and found there was not a listing. The Marketing Director also checked with the Department of Insurance to see if this Stoploss carrier was admitted. The results from the DOI there was no an admitted carrier in the jurisdiction. The Marketing Director did due diligence based on the agreements the TPA uses with Plan Sponsors on using on A rated or better companies with AM Best. The Marketing Director called the owner of the TPA and relayed the findings. The owner said to continue in requesting the quote as this underwriter /stoploss carrier was the same as Lloyds of London and would not be shown by AM Best.

The quotes came in and were processed in a spreadsheet for Agent 1. The quotes were very competitive and the new underwriter/Stoploss carrier quotes was the lowest, even lower than the current rates of the Plan Sponsor. Agent 1 was informed of the new underwriter / Stoploss carrier not being rated by AM Best and was not an admitted carrier in the jurisdiction of the DOI (Department of Insurance). Agent 1 determined to utilize the quote of the new underwriter / Stoploss carrier. Agent 1 requested changes to the quotation of vendor fees and Stoploss commissions.

Modifying the Quote

Agent 1 wanted to modify the quote to make as much money as he was making under the current program used by the plan sponsor. The Marketing Director asked how he would like to modify the vendor costs and Stoploss. Agent 1 stated he would like to add $4.00 PEPM (Per Employee Per Month) to the Administration Fees taking the fees from $21.00 PEPM to $25.00 PEPM. Additionally, Agent 1 wanted a Broker Compensation Fee of $2.00 PEPM which was disclosed in the quote to the Plan Sponsor. The Marketing Director stated he could not add fees to the Plan Administration Fee as this additional fee must be disclosed to the Plan Sponsor. Agent 1 replied that he did not want the Plan Sponsor to know how much he was making and the inclusion in the Administrative Fees would not show on the 5500 Form for his fees. Agent 1 called the owner of the TPA and stated what he wanted to do and handed the phone to the Marketing Director which explained the conversation with Agent 1. The TPA owner said do what Agent 1 was wanting. Additionally, Agent 1 requested the Stoploss commissions be at 10%. The Marketing Director did as requested. Agent 1 requested the commissions be paid to the TPA and for the TPA to write the check to agent 1 and to not disclose the amount to the Plan Sponsor.

Quote was prepared as requested for Agent 1 to present with the statement from the Marketing Director attached: *The quote attached is reinsured with The.....Trust. This is the same status as Lloyds of London. Neither of these organizations are rated by AM Best.*

The following is an email from the Marketing Director to Agent 1 used in discovery:

"In following up on our conversation earlier this evening, Owner - President of TPA directed me as an employee of his firm to include Underwriter/ stoploss in the quoting process. Prior to his phone call to me, when I was an employee, I had never heard of Underwriter/Stoploss. In addition, you and I had a conversation on this in 2010 which the same was stated. Per a follow up conversation between you and I, you confirmed this information from a discussion you had with Owner - President of TPA where he stated yes he told me to use United Re in the quoting process. I hope this clears up any confusion as to where the contact and direction came from on the inclusion of Underwriter/stoploss in the quoting process for TPA.'

It is important to understand the above inorder to grasp the direction of the TPA Owner and Agent 1 to use the New Underwriter/Stoploss which created a significant issue for the Plan and Plan Sponsor.

This case is based on a complaint by the Plan Sponsor regarding the non-reimbursement of claims covered under the Stoploss agreement / trust. Thus, the TPA (Owner and Marketing Director), Stoploss carrier, and Agent 1 we named in the complaint. The TPA Marketing Director terminated employment on 7/2009. This is important as the complaint regarding these issues occured 2/2010 regarding a default of payment by the Underwriter/Stoploss Carrier of approximately $900,000+ from the 2009 plan year. Also important is that the TPA and Agent 1 and Plan Sponsor renewed with the Underwriter/ Stoploss carrier for 2010 and the Marketing Director was not involved. This is significant as the Plan Sponsor renewed the agreements with the TPA, Agent 1 and Underwriter/Stoploss for the 2010 stop/loss policy.

As stated in the previous chapters - everything is discoverable - having the knowledge and how to utilize proper analytical tools provides the means to uncover the objective facts. The previous chapters have prepared you to discover the objective facts.

Review of Agents

Agent 1 was the initiator of the case at hand with the plan sponsor. Upon investigation, Agent 1 had significant issues that arose during the initial plan year with the DOI. The DOJ found Agent 1 guilty of Fraud regarding to the false statements on the number of employees to obtain a lower premium. This was reviewed nationally and several DOI's in their jurisdiction terminated the License of Agent 1. Agent 1 directed payments of fees and commissions to be made to Agent 2, information provided to the TPA with a copy of Agent 2 license and TIN. All payments were made going forward to Agent 2 in February 2009. Upon review of Agent 2 was properly licensed with the DOI in the jurisdiction; therefore, Agent 2 was not part of the complaint filed by the Plan Sponsor.

Review of TPA

The TPA was appropriately licensed by the DOI in their jurisdiction. The TPA and Owner of the TPA made an agreement with the Underwriter / Stoploss carrier in receiving 5% of the premiums generated by the TPA with Underwriter / Stoploss carrier. This agreement was not known by the Marketing Director prior to the termination in 7/2009. This was brought forth in discovery on a monetary exchange between the TPA and the Underwriter / Stoploss Carrier.

The TPA and Marketing Director provided the appropriate information to the Underwriter / Stoploss Carrier with regard to the Plan and Plan Sponsor for the RFQ (Request for Quote). The paperwork was completed in its entirety with the disclosure form completed in detail. The only finding was the TPA added Commission to the rates quoted by the Underwriter / Stoploss carrier without notification to adjust the quote and proper calculation of the Surplus line and municipal taxes. This is a basis for Insurance Fraud.

The TPA in review processed the claims appropriately for the Plan and Plan Sponsor as well as with the Administrative Service Agreement for the Plan / Plan Sponsor. The TPA appropriately filed the claims with the underwriter / plan sponsor on a timely basis and processed the premium payments from the Plan Sponsors Health Plan Account on a timely basis.

The question which arose was the financial agreement between the TPA and Owner with the Underwriter / Stoploss carrier. On the surface this looks like a bias to do business with the parties to this arrangement. Additionally, the findings showed the TPA processed the payments to the Underwriter / Stoploss company after reducing the agent commissions. It is not known if the agreement between the TPA and Underwriter / Stoploss was paid out based on the 5%. The 5% was not disclosed to the Plan Sponsor as well as other fees paid to the Agents. There was a responsibility by the TPA and Agents to disclose these fees to the Plan Sponsor. This could be a basis for fraud by not disclosing to the Fiduciary of the Plan - Plan Sponsor. Additionally, the addition of the commission by the TPA on the Stoploss rates to the plan and not calculating the appropriate taxes to the DOI for Surplus Lines Tax and Municipal Tax is a basis for Fraud on several counts - tax avoidance and changing the rates in an insurance quote without notification to the insurance company.

Review of Underwriter / Stoploss Carrier

The underwriter / Stoploss carrier upon review was not admitted by the DOI in their jurisdiction for the plan. Additionally, this was considered a Trust and the effective insuring organization was off shore and not admitted by any DOI of the United States of America. This organization filed under Chapter 11 in protection. A statement was uncovered in a memo to the TPA that the TPA did not notify Agent 1 or Agent 2 or the Plan / Plan Sponsor of the information in the Memo. This is significant as the TPA had knowledge which must be communicated to the Fiduciaries of the Plan. By the TPA having knowledge of this the view of culpability is raised in the Complaint by the Plan Sponsor to hold the TPA responsible for the unpaid reimbursement by the Underwriter / Stoploss carrier, even though the TPA filed appropriately for the reimbursement of the excess claims to the Underwriter / Stoploss carrier.

The objective fact was the TPA had knowledge of the status of the Underwriter / Stoploss Carrier (non admitted carrier with DOI in jurisdiction and Chapter 11 filing). The TPA had knowledge of the filings made on behalf of the Plan / Plan Sponsor for reimbursement of the $900,000+. The TPA had knowledge of adding to the Stoploss insurance quote for the commissions to the agent and avoiding the additional cost for surplus lines and municipal taxes. Therefore, the case is a culpability of the TPA in regard to the claims and complaint sby the Plan / Plan Sponsor.

Review of Plan Sponsor

The Plan Sponsor is a longtime employer in the community. They have used Agent 1 services for many years. The Plan Sponsor made the decision to go with the self funded plan using the underwriter / Stoploss carrier presented by Agent 1 with the disclosure on the quote: ***The quote attached is reinsured with The.....Trust. This is the same status as Lloyds of London. Neither of these organizations are rated by AM***

Best. This is an objective fact and the Plan / Plan Sponsor was informed of the status of the Underwriter / Stoploss Carrier. The quotes shown by Agent 1 to the Plan and Plan Sponsor only showed one of the many Stoploss quotes provided by the TPA to Agent 1. Agent 1, in his sole discretion, decided to show only one self funded quote to the Plan / Plan Sponsor, but showed four 4 quotes on the fully insured side. The quote presented by Agent 1 showed the increase in the Stoploss premiums by the addition of the 10% commission. In review of the Underwriter / Stoploss agreement, it was presented without the increase in cost by the addition of the 10% commission. The company signed off on the agreement and trust with the net cost of the premiums.

The objective facts are Agent 1 presented the quote with the additional cost included in the premiums and did not disclose the difference to the Plan / Plan Sponsor. Agent 1 did not disclose the additional $4.00 PEPM fees added to the Administrative Fees to the Plan / Plan Sponsor. The discloser was made on the $2.00 PEPM on the Broker Compensation Fee. The Plan / Plan Sponsor as the Fiduciary has the right to full disclosure and any compensation paid by the Vendors to the Plan. Agent 1 is culpable of Insurance Fraud, and Fraud to the Plan in non disclosure of added compensation and avoidance of information reported on Form 5500 Schedule A.

Review of information from the PBM (Prescription Benefit Management Company) revealed rebates had been paid to the plan. The Plan Sponsor did not apply the rebates to the Health Plan Account. This is significant as the rebates are owned by the Plan as refunds and ultimately are used to offset the Aggregate claims to the plan. The rebates from the PBM totaled $16,105.25. These rebates are used to reduce the Aggregate which includes the request for reimbursement on the claims exceeding the Aggregate Attachment Point for the Plan. Not including this reduction can be considered a fraud to the insurance company for a false filing for an excess gain to the plan.

Review of 5500 Form for 2009 and 2010 revealed the Plan / Plan Sponsor did not complete the form and related schedules with regard to the self funded plan. The objective facts provided the Plan / Plan Sponsor had been filing 5500 Forms and the appropriate Schedules for years but did not file the appropriate information with regard to the 2009 and 2010 plan years. It appears this was intentional by the Plan / Plan Sponsor. This was discovered and it wassuggested the Plan Sponsor amend and file appropriately. There are significant fines for not filing the appropriate information with regard to 5500 Forms and related schedules when done intentionally.

This scenario utilized many of the tools discussed in this book. Normally, cases are not as intricate as this one. To get through a case like this it is important to have a methodology and process utilizing the proper algorithms and analytics. This provides a scientific basis for duplication of the objective facts without subjective interference. The process of critical thinking to look beyond the obvious and dig deeper to discover the objective facts provides a basis for truth and the mechanism to write a great factual report.

There are many other types of Fraud with regard to health plans such as billing, up charging, unbundling of claims. Let's look at a scenario of a Hospitalist to observe billing fraud. This is broken down in different incidents to provide a basis for viewing how this can occur. A Hospitalist in these scenarios are physicians.

Hospitalist Scenario One

Hospitalist billing multiple times for the same time period on multiple patients. The average time spent by a hospitalist is 4.5 minutes per patient. In a case reviewed the hospitalist was averaging about $338 per patient visit. Lets look at this in perspective. In one hour, the Hospitalist would see approximately 12 patients. The billing for this was in total $4,056 for the hour. This breaks down to $67.60 per minute. The base salary on average is about $250,000 per year. If broken down by hour using 2080 hours per year is about $120.19 per hour. The above billing would provide approximately $8,436,480 per year using a 2080 hours per year and the $4056 per hour as shown above for billing. This is excessive. In review, billing records per day were requested with detail for time spent per patient. The times did not match up as the hospitalist could not be in three places at the same time.

Hospitalist Scenario Two (Actual Case)

This scenario is a sceme used to get the most amount of money from the patient due to the basis for in-network deductible and out-of-pocket maximum vs a separate out-of-network deductible and out-of-pocket maximum. This sceme is used to maximize fees to the hospitalist but penalizes the patient/member due to increaed out-of-pocket costs. The patient had no choice of hospitalist as the patient was in an in-network hospital. The following are the findings.

Review of a patient bill from a hospitalist organization shows *two distinct billings* from *two hospitalist* in the **same organization in-network**. Hospitalist One is *in the PPO Network* while Hospitalist Two is **not in the PPO Network** even though their *organization is listed in-network*. The *hospital is in-network* with the PPO. The patient had no choice of who was seeing them in the hospital. The billing for a patient seen two times in two days resulted in the following:

The following are facts to this case which are as follow:

Patient incurred an acute condition which sent her to the emergency room at the XYZ Hospital. Patient was put in a room for observation at XYZ Hospital. The initial care took place on 1/24/2016 with code 99222 and was discharged on 1/25/2016 with Code 99238.

Claims were filed to the Health Plan Carrier.

The maximum in-network out-of-pocket maximum was met and subsequently the Patient paid their responsibility.

CLAIMS FILED BY: Dr. One / XXX Hospital

Health Plan Carrier claim numbers:

Claim ID 16034F0XXXXX was filed on 01/24/2016 in the amount of $346.00.
Claim ID 16040EAXXXXX was filed on 01/25/2016 in the amount of $185.00.

Total: $ 531.00

These claims were subsequently turned over to a collections company: XXX health; PO Box 12345, City, State 12345-6789. Ph: 888-432-xxxx.

Patient made calls to XXX health:

Timelines intentionally left out for this scenario

With the above timeline, information and facts, XXX health and Dr. One with XYZ Hospital have created a problem for patient. Non-compliance from XXX health and Dr. One with XYZ Hospital on requests for corrected claims reflecting the proper location and Point of Service (POS) have been ignored.

By the implied willful non-compliance by each XXX health and Dr. One with XXX Hospital has the appearance of fraud. From the date of the first request for the corrected claims to the date of this report July 25, 2016 provided ample time for the corrected claims to have been submitted to Health Plan Carrier for proper processing and payment.

Recommendations:

Patient not to remit any funds as the validity of the claim made is based on errors and inconsistency with location and point of service. Additionally, patient has met her out-of-pocket maximum and remitted the out of pocket to the proper providers in full.

Remove any and all collection processes in regard to the above mentioned claims by XXX health and Dr. One - Claim ID 16040EAXXXX and Dr. Two - Claim ID 16034F0CXXXX with XYZ Hospital on Patient.

Due to the objective facts and circumstances above this bill was written off.

Summary: These are schemes utilized by healthcare providers to receive the most amount of money to the detriment of the patient financially. This happens within many disciplines in the healthcare fields. When these schemes are discovered and confronted with the facts, the organizations involved will normally waive the fees to avoid an issue with federal organization coming in and auditing their billing practices.

If the above recommendations are not completed:

A request for an investigation on each XXX health and Dr. One with XYZ Hospital for possible billing fraud to an Insurance / Health Plan. Referred to the Attorney General Office of the Commonwealth of Kentucky, Commonwealth of Kentucky Department of Insurance Fraud Division.

Request the Health Plan Carrier SIU review all claims submitted from Dr. One and Dr. Two with XYZ Hospital for possible billing fraud.

Dr. One and Dr. Two report to the Kentucky Medical Association and XYZ Hospital to Kentucky Hospital Association for review of non compliance with a health plan request on claims to be filed correctly with the specific areas to be corrected in a timely manner and possible basis for fraud.

Respectfully Submitted,

The Examiner

Result

Claim on patient paid in full by Health Plan Carrier with reduction for discounts. Dr. One and Dr. Two accepted payment as payment in full. Helping people navigate the complexity of this type of case is very rewarding.

Hospitalist Scenario Three

Patient is billed and hospitalist is not in-network but is providing services at an in-network hospital. Patient assumes all incurred claims will be in-network. Patient has no choice of Hospitalist. The following is a result of working through the facts and rfinding a resolution. This was the letter sent to…and results were accepted by the billing entity.

Dear XXX,

I'm concerned that the communication within your firm XXXX Management Systems regarding the $343.00 has not been conveyed to you from John Doe EE# 625 ph 866-767-XXXX via a conversation disputing in full this claim. On 6/22/2017 communication via telephone with the above mentioned individual and subsequently with Ms. Smith from XXXX Management Systems took place via conversation with Health Plan Carrier on Claim from XYZ Hospital - Dr. One was being reprocessed as in-network by Health Plan Carrier and payment of $130.82 would be forthcoming and allow 30 days for processing from June 22, 2017 and should be completed by August 3, 2017 per Health Plan Carrier. The balance of the $212.18 is what Health Plan Carrier considers the discount for in-network services as the services were provided at an in network facility. As the patient had no other options made available to them nor did Dr. One notify patient prior to treatment that he was **not** in-network. Thus, all services would be considered as in-network. This should be considered closed and paid in full when check is received by Health Plan Carrier.

If there is further harassment regarding this issue by your firm to the patient, patient will have no other choice but to bring in legal counsel and take action against XXXX Management Systems, XXX Health, XYZ Hospital and Dr. One.

Respectfully Submitted,
The Examiner

Result

Claim on patient was paid in full by Health Plan Carrier with reduction for discounts. Dr. One accepted payment as payment in full.

These are just a few of the types of claims that could be considered for Fraud. In the above scenarios one of the Dr.'s was in-network and the other Dr. was out-of-network, both working for the same company and providing services at an in-network facility. Many times, this scenario exists to increase the billing to the company as the out-of-network Dr. can balance bill the patient for the difference not allowed by the Health Plan Carrier. Remember the Patient did not have a choice and thought the providers providing services at the in-network facility are in-network. When investigating it is likely to find this scenario and should be considered for resolve from above scenarios or given to the appropriate agencies for investigation.

Fraud and Eye Doctors (Actual Case)

During an eye exam the Dr. stated he needed to ruse a testing instrument that took pictures of the retina. The Dr. stated he would have to bill the medical insurance on this procedure instead of billing the Dental Insurance which also carried the Vision Coverage. Previously, the patient's husband had the same eye exam with the same instrument, the same medical insurance and dental insurance and the cost was $40.

The Dr. provided the same analysis as was done on the patient. The underlying issue with this is the Dr. billed the health insurance provider $299 for this procedure. With this patient having a high deductible plan, this would be 100% out of pocket cost. It must be noted the Dr. stated the same to the spouse and the spouse asked what the cash price was and it was stated $40. The spouse has a potential medical condition RP which must be looked at each exam due to the father having RP.

The Dr. was approached and this billing practice was discussed with the office manager regarding the up charging by stating this was a medical procedure and must be billed to the health plan. The perception of fraud with this type of billing practice was noted. The Dr. and the office manager stated the patient did not have to pay anything and retracted the billing. This Dr. now does the procedure for the $40.

The above various scenarios and discussion only touch the surface of how fraud can be committed. When documenting the objective findings, be prepared to document how the client can put in safeguards and policies to reduce or eliminate fraud.

Utilizing the Forensic Decision Mapping Algorithm for each of the above descriptions of potential fraud will provide the basis to collect the objective facts for solving the various class of problems listed. The reasoning and methodology of the forensic decision mapping process will provide the unambiguous specifications of how to solve the issues at hand. This basis of critical thinking structures the flow to obtain the objective facts and explain how they were uncovered.

Money Laundering

Money Laundering has become an important issue since September 11, 2001 due to the terrorist attacks on the United States. Controls were put in place due the fact that laundered money financed many of the pre-attack preparations. It is important to understand how the cleansing of money can be accomplished by using a self-funded health plan. The proper structured systematic focus on money and the distribution of money through a means that allows for dirty money to become cleansed or "laundered".

There are many methods and schemes to be used in order to accomplish the goal of cleansed money. The tracking of the transactions can be difficult. The use of the Forensic Decision Mapping Algorithm can help to trace and catch the launderers. In this chapter we will discuss some scenarios which when done properly in the structure will have the perception of a legitimate business when in fact it is only a cover and sometimes has the element of both legal and illegal factors. These businesses may have their operational structures separated from the legal ones for laundering and payments to the support organization as well as the distribution to the various cells contained within the United States and abroad.

Those who need to clean their money understand there is a cost to structure the process and they accept it. The one thing that usually catches the organization and leads to thier down fall is a term used in my first book: Forensics of a Medical Plan - Dissecting Health Benefits on a Company Level - and that is the **G- Factor,** also known as the **Greed Factor.**

Let's first understand the following definitions and methods.

Organized Crime Defined

The FBI defines organized crime as any group having some manner of a formalized structure and whose primary objective is to obtain money through illegal activities. Such groups maintain their position through the use of actual or threatened violence, corrupt public officials, graft, or extortion, and generally have a significant impact on the people in their locales, region, or the country as a whole.

Do you have a definition you use?

Money laundering is defined as the process of concealing or disguising the proceeds of a crime or converting those proceeds into goods and services. It allows criminals to infuse money obtained illegally into the stream of commerce, thus corrupting financial institutions and the money supply. While many definitions for money laundering exist, it can be defined very simply as any knowing use of the proceeds of criminal activity.

Money laundering is usually associated with crimes that provide a financial gain. This includes, but is not limited to, bank fraud, insurance fraud, mortgage fraud, health care fraud, securities/commodities frauds, advanced fee schemes, high yield and prime bank note schemes, Ponzi schemes, government fraud, corporate and occupational frauds, cyber crimes, public corruption, drugs, organized crime, and the financing of terrorism. Money laundering differs from other types of criminal acts in that it is not a stand-alone crime. The laundering of funds is typically a secondary criminal act – typically without proceeds from an underlying crime, there can be no money laundering.

Money Laundering Methods

The number and variety of methods used by criminals to launder money render it impossible to provide a complete listing. The means to launder money is limited only by the creativity and ability of the launderers. Increasingly, new technology provides ever more avenues for criminals to launder money. The FBI works with its international, federal, state and local partners to identify and combat new money laundering methods as they emerge.

The use of money derived from illegal activity by concealing the identity of the individuals who obtained the money and converting it to assets that appear to have come from a legitimate source is the objective of the money launderer.

Source: Money Laundering - A Guide for Criminal Investigators - Third Edition. John Madinger.

The money laundering cycle includes three stages: placement, layering and integration.

How would you describe each cycle of money laundering?

Placement

Placement- involves either the conversion of currency into some other form or the physical movement of the currency. Placement of dirty money relies on businesses that deal heavily in cash, as well as all types of financial institutions.

Layering

Layering - attempting to hide their tracks on the paper trail. Layers of transactions, business entities, fronts, or other concealment mechanisms are imposed between the money and its source.

Integration

Integration - uses the same financial institutions and instruments employed in placement and layering thereby making the funds look as if their origin is legitimate, resulting in some really creative schemes.

How would you describe a Money Launderer?

The Money Launderer is like a magician, who uses proven and secret techniques to make obtained dirty money moved to what appears to be legitament operations.

Why is Flexibility important?

Flexibility is a key to the money launderer for success in money laundering operations.

What is the Key objective for the Money Launderer?

Money laundering as a cycle, the objective is to have access to "clean" appearing money at the end of the process. The recipient does not care how their money was cleansed but that it is done.

Let's take a look at how currency smuggling is accomplished from the following matrix. This will provide a means for tracking as the launderer wants to make it difficult as funds can be converted to other hard assets such as vehicles and property.

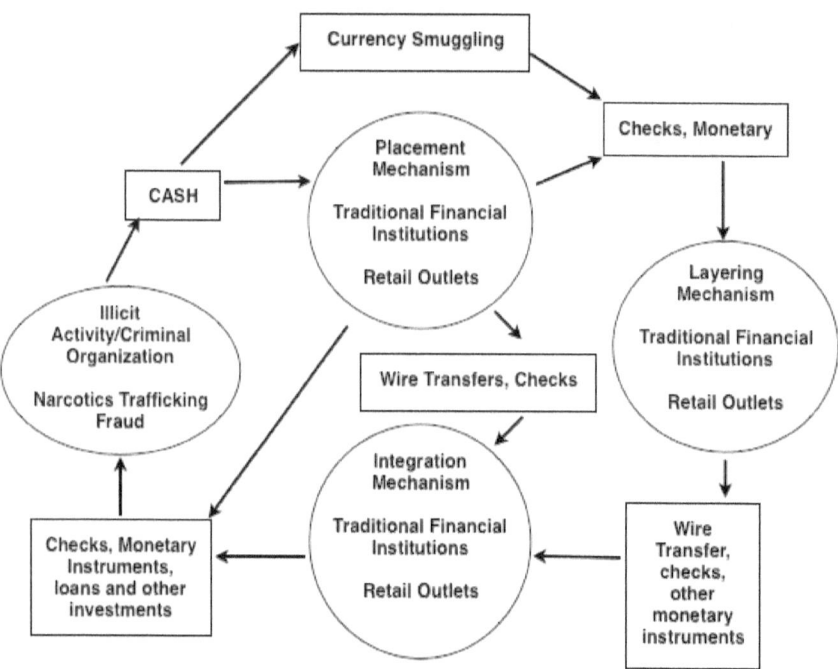

With the following schemes, Phase 1 and Phase 2, we will look at the structure based on the three stages of Money Laundering. Since this involves self funded health plans, it is important to understand the self funded health plan and its vendor architecture and why the Organized Crime Syndicates would choose this structure to accomplish the result for the appearance of Clean Money.

There are three stages to laundering money: placement, layering and integration. There are many ways to launder money but we will specifically refer to to Self-Funded Health Plans.

Background

This brief backgroundwill provide a setup to how and why organized crime may choose to utilize an administrator to launder money through a self-funded health plan. When this author had a TPA it actually had two sets of the same software — one for operations and the second for training and preprocessing updates to make sure the update was good.

The updates when proven good would then update the production/operation "live" system. With this information, it would allow for an administrator to process off of the training system independently.

Banking

Most banking institutions do not look at the health plan accounts as they do other accounts. Health plans will typically receive deposits for the month in excess of $10,000 and will write payments for $10,000 or more either to pay contracted vendors to the plan or providers and institutions for medical services. As an example the TPA, had clients ranging in size from 25 to over 2000 employee lives. A group of 1600 lives was depositing approximately $16,000,000+ per year in their health plan account.

Account setup normally utilized for the laundering is an FBO account structured by the TPA. With a TPA that has had a relationship with a bank for years this becomes the norm and is an easy structure to set up. Banks are happy to receive the funds.

Cost

Organized crime accepts the cost to launder money as normal in a business transaction. The organized crime pays a TPA for services to help in laundering the money. The cost charged by the TPA will be more than the normal PEPM fees. If a TPA was charging $25 PEPM for legitimate business it may charge $50 for the laundering process so on a 1600 employee group the monthly fee would be approximately $80,000 or $960,000 annually. This is usually about 5% to 10% of the total amount to launder.

Case Scenario

A criminal organization is looking how to structure their money from drug, weapons and human trafficking, etc. They have large sums of funds to launder. The organization knows an individual that owns a Third Party Administration (TPA) firm. The owner of the TPA is invited to a dinner meeting by the individual who is the head of the organization looking to structure their money and get it cleaned. The discussion may go as follow: They discuss the operational structure of the TPA and the current volume of funds flowing through the self funded plans at the bank the TPA uses for their administrative accounts for their clients. The owner of the TPA is proud that they have a training system which is exactly the same as their live operational system. The TPA states the system is used to train our employees how to set up plans, plan sponsors, process and adjudicate claims, and process the payments to vendors to the plan as well as payments to providers. The TPA owner states this system is also used to process any updates received from the software company prior to updating their operational live system to catch errors and have them corrected. The head of the organization looking to clean their funds tells the owner of the TPA he has a client they want to put under the training system and have the account set up by the TPA as an FBO account for the health plan. It is stated there will be about 1600 individuals on the plan. The head of the organization states he has his own vendors to set up for the plan and their own network of providers. He would like a three year agreement. The price for the PEPM will be $50.00 so the fee to the TPA will be about $80,000 per month or $960,000 per year. He would like to have two of their people trained to operate the medical plan administration for this client using the TPAs software system. He states these individuals will be paid by their organization directly and the TPA does not have to pay them a salary. The TPA asked about the volume of dollars from this account to go through the FBO account at the bank. The head of the organization states it would be between $16,000,000 and $20,000,000 not including the rebates from the prescriptions, reimbursements from Stoploss or other contributions. The TPA asks when do they want this plan to begin. The head of the organization wants to go live in 60 days. The TPA says they will need a set up fee to get everything done in 60 days. The head of the organization states they will pay one month of $80,000 as a set up fee. An agreement is reached.

The head of the organization introduces the two individuals who will be trained. The TPA establishes the FBO account at the bank and tells the bank this will be a large client and will have approximately $1.3 to $1.6 million deposited per month and the organization will have the money wired directly to the account. The head of the organization provides the information on the vendors to the plan to be paid with the pepm. Note: the vendors are locations the organization supports, they will have the name of the companies and address to write the checks to. As far as the EIN's in the training system for payments, those will be made up/bogus since there will not be any 1099s issued from the plan to vendors or providers as all of those individuals/entities are part of the organization. So the break out of vendors is as follows:

Third Party Administrator - (The TPA which agreed to this structure)
Stoploss - Organization location 1
PPO Network - Organization location 2
Managed Care Company - Organization location 3
Aggregator - Organization location 4
PBM - Organization location 5
Consultant - Organization location 6
Insurance Agency - Organization location 7
(Additional vendors can be added as the organization needs)
(Each of the organization locations above will establish an account at the bank. Each of these locations will be using different banks as this makes it more difficult to track the money. These Locations are considered "Mules" as a pass through for the funds).

As an examiner, this is the time to set up the Forensic Decision Mapping on a MACRO level and with the ability to track on the MICRO level to capture details.

Now that all is in place and set up, the process starts. (Remember, the organization stated this was to run for three years).

The first deposit is wired to the bank for the FBO account. The first is a test to make sure all goes well. Once confirmed and posted, the second level of transactions for laundering starts by making payments to the vendors with checks for the TPA and locations 1 - 7.

These checks are cut from a **micr** system and **micr** printer tied to the training system utilizing blank check stock. (Blank check stock is used as to not have check stock with routing and account information in a physical instrument. This would be important if an FBO account was not used.) NOTE: The FBO Account ties to the Third Party Administrator not the Organization.

If the organization did not want to write checks, then ACHs or Virtual Checks could be issued. In some cases, the payments and/or physical checks may be issued/sent to a lock box and instructions for transferring the funds to other accounts may be part of the instructions for the Lock Box agreement. If a Lock Box is used then this electronic transaction can be a third level for distribution to other accounts.

Claims are generated for other locations of the organization which are set up to print and mail. These will usually be done US Mail or Fax. There will be a fax machine with a separate number from that of the TPAs regular Fax Machine or may be picked up by the computer and then processed by using a split screen. The claims received will not have a physical basis but only a virtual one that exists in the Training System. This is important to keep separated from the TPA production system as the agreement is for three years to use the training system. Payments are made from the processing of the claims and sent as printed from the micr system, ACH or use of a virtual check. Additionally, these payments may be made to a lock box with instructions.

Transactions from the lock box and the distribution of the funds creates another level of cleansing the money.

Two of the vendors, Stoploss and PBM to the plan have a basis for depositing funds to the FBO Account as well. This provides another avenue for the organization to launder money. Since there is no actual Stoploss insurance on this scenario plan, a Stoploss reimbursement can be made at anytime to the plan if the Organization finds it needs to launder additional monies. These can be substantial transactions anywhere from a few thousand dollars to a million plus. The PBM can also make a deposit due to declaring there are rebates due the plan to launder additional monies.

There are many variations, different scenarios and schemes for investing in legitimate businesses, such as the market for investments, purchasing cars, property or many other areas where money could be "cleaned".

The object of this scenario is to show how money laundering can be accomplished. Remember the agreement for three years? If held to three years, the data from this case would be deleted and cleansed from the system. The Organization may decide to buy the TPA a new Training system with hardware and completely destroy the old system. But, due to the G-Factor and the ease of this type and level of laundering the Organization may continue. This is what normally catches the Organization and brings it down.

The Forensic Practitioner can recognize the potential for money laundering and provide the decision mapping which when properly done will show where the money came from and went based on the mapping structure. This scenario shows the overall structure for the placement, layering and integration of the dirty money to clean / laundered money. There are many additional details in structuring this type of laundering. At times the "Mules" will get greedy or mad since they feel they should be receiving more money. They may be the ones who are considered the thread to unravel the organization by being the informant.

By using the training system for this scenario, an auditor will approach the main operating system and software to find the money in an audit.

The Auditor will only find legitimate business on the operation system and normally may never look at the training system for the transactions.

The following shows this can be duplicated for multiple false plans.

Money Laundering Decision Mapping

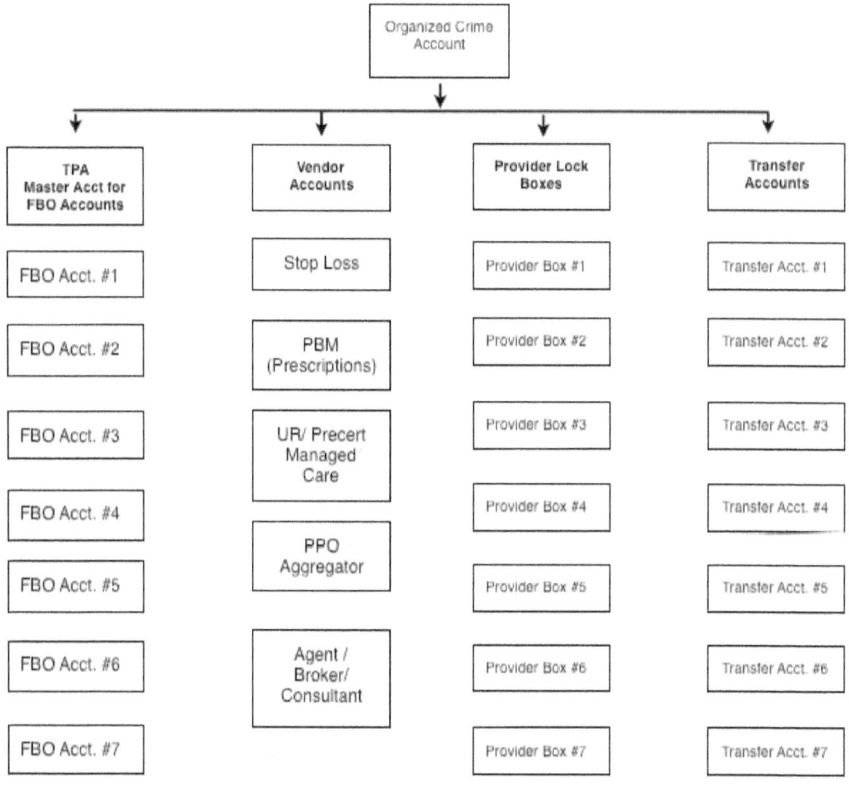

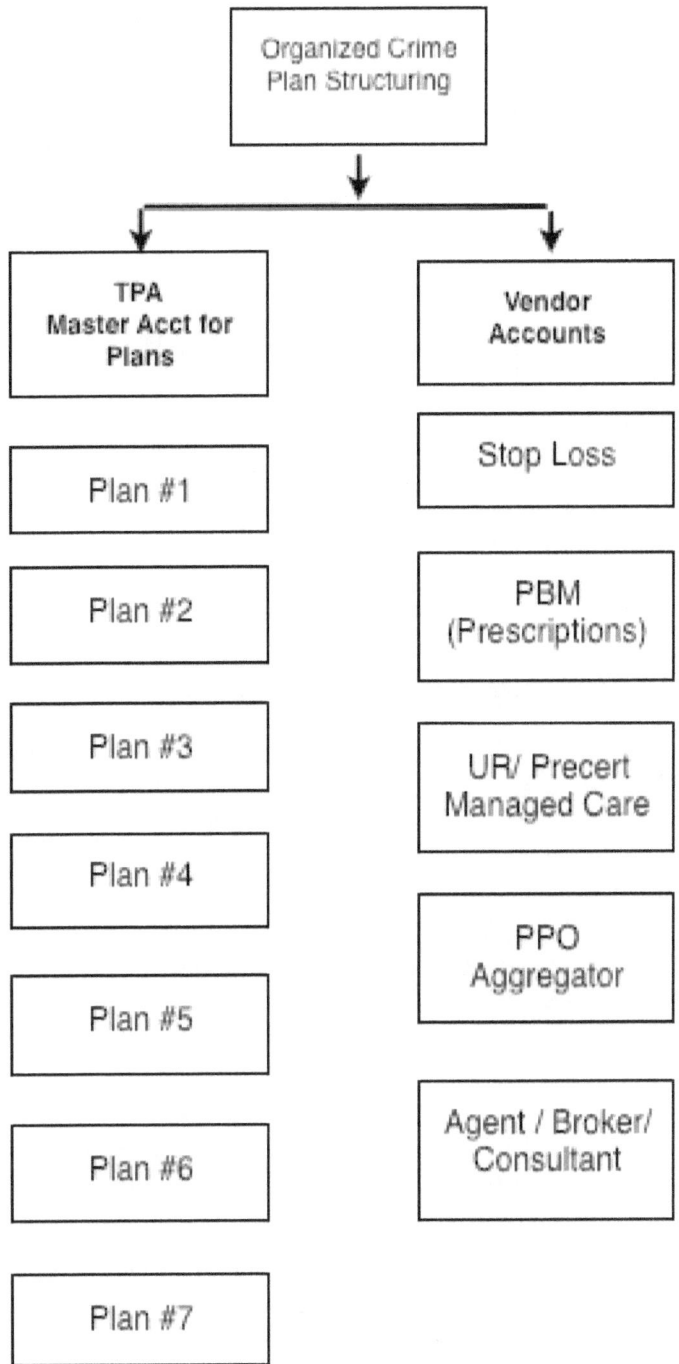

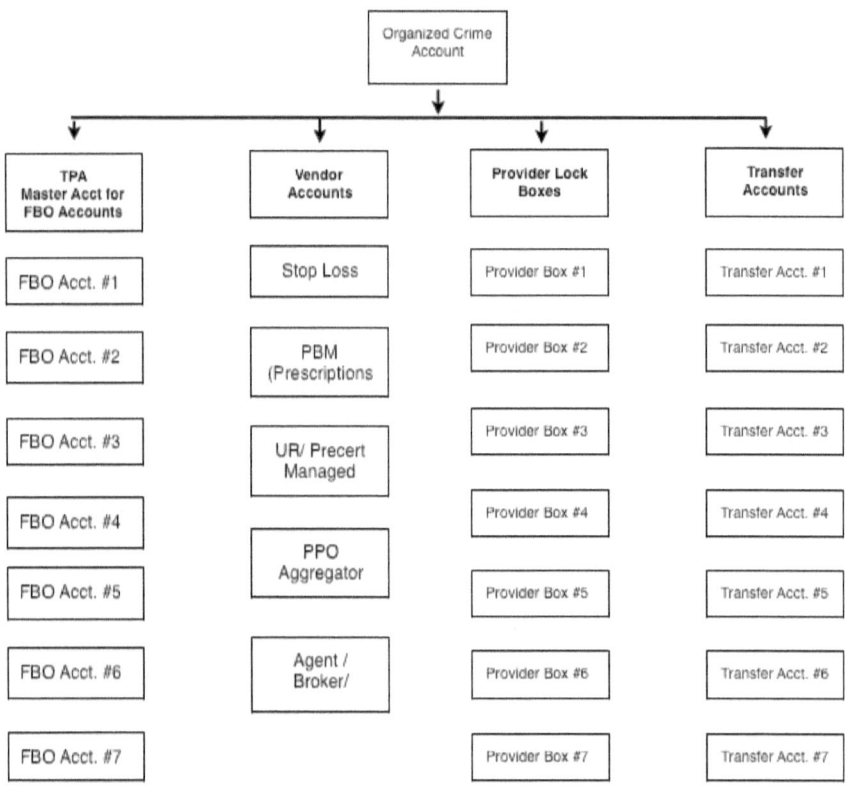

IBNR and IRBNP

The following is from a case that involved two Third Party Contracted Administrators. Information has been modified in the report for privacy requirements regarding the Plan Sponsor, Members of the Health Plan and names of the Contracted Third Party Administration firms involved. The report will provide the structure for how the investigation, gathering the objective facts and evidence and the conclusion to the issue at hand was documented. Every circumstance you will encounter as a forensic analyst will be different and require the basis for critical thinking and not regurgitative thinking. All work is unique to the issue and situation at hand. This report will bring in the level of analytics that have been covered in this book.

This case involved IRBNP (Incurred Received But Not Processed) claims. This is significant when there is a specific or aggregate issue for reimbursement. IBNR (Incurred But Not Received) claims are addressed as well in the report.

FORENSIC ANALYSIS AND REPORT
IRBNP

Plan Sponsor Health Benefit Plan

2011, 2012, 2013, 2014 Plan Years

F. Randall Childers, Jr., CFC, DABFE
ACFEI - Certified Forensic Consultant
(Speciality - Self Funded Health Benefit Plans)

Completed Report Date: 1 November 2014

I reserve the right to change, modify or correct any and all comments or conclusions expressed in my written observations should I be given additional information that would warrant such actions.

Overview

The following will detail the claims for reimbursement from TPA 1 as well as the circumstances which create the claims from Plan Sponsor Medical Plan.

The forensic report utilized an analytical comparison of the data provided and the agreements provided on the vendor architecture of the plan. The vendors to the plan each provided a specific area of expertise in the function of the Plan Sponsor Health Benefit Plan. This plan is a self funded plan utilizing Stoploss insurance as a protection to the health benefit plan from a risk basis in protecting the cash flow due to large claims on both a specific and aggregate protection level.

This report is designed to show the findings of the health benefit plan forensic analysis. Forensic practice in Health Benefits remains completely objective in making an accurate determination of the facts involved and the presentation of the facts.

Note: TPA 1 assets were acquired by Maxor Plan Administrators, LLC effective for January 1, 2014. TPA 1 was responsible for processing all health and prescription claims and filing all request for reimbursements for specific and or aggregate Stoploss through Tuesday, December 31, 2014.

I reserve the right to change, modify or correct any and all comments or conclusions expressed in my written observations should I be given additional information that would warrant such actions.

The **first level** is based on the claims as processed by TPA 1 and the application of Stoploss filings which were not done by TPA 1 in the normal course of providing administrative services pursuant to:

III. Duties of TPA 1

3.2 **Claim Services**
3,2,1 Services
3.2.1.10 Use its best efforts in the normal course of its services hereunder to identify claims that may be subject to reimbursement, based upon the existence of any Stoploss or Reinsurance Policy. In no event will TPA 1 be held liable for any claims not covered or not paid by the Stoploss or Reinsurance Carrier.

(See Exhibit A - Administration Agreement)

The **second level** is based on the "IBNR" and extracted "IRBNP" claims.

The forensic analytics are applied for IBNR (incurred but not received) and IRBNP (incurred received but not processed)

IBNR are claims incurred in the previous plan year but not received or processed in the previous plan year. These are normally due to a LAG (time frame for incurred claims but not filed for reimbursement by the providers for payment of claims.

IRBNP (incurred received but not processed) are claims incurred and filed by the providers and received by the contracted administrator but not processed in a timely manner by the contracted administrator in the appropriate plan year for Stoploss contracts.

The contracts for Stoploss are two fold: Specific Stoploss based on a 15/12 contract for claims incurred from October 1 in the previous plan year and paid in the current year January 1 to December 31. Aggregate Stoploss is based on a 12/12 contract for claims which is incurred January 1 of the current year and paid by December 31 of the current plan year.

Both IBNR and IRBNP claims have application to Stoploss contracts whether in the current plan year or previous plan year. The application of these claims are dependent on the Stoploss contract provisions of incurred and paid. Some claims may not have an application to the Stoploss contract based on incurred date of claims as well as processed date of claims submitted by providers and the processing by the contracted administrator.

SUMMARY TOTALS JANUARY 2014 TO DECEMBER 31, 2014 SPECIFIC Stoploss ANALYSIS					
Name	Claims Pd	Spec Stoploss	Over Spec	Amount Reimb.	Amount Due Plan
5	$7,624.24	$25,000.00		$0.00	
1	$109,773.49	$35,000.00	$74,773.49	$74,296.62	$476.87
7	$38,933.51	$40,000.00		$0.00	
11	$2,124.98	$40,000.00		$0.00	
12	$53,880.40	$40,000.00	$13,880.40	$11,856.08	$2,024.32
18	$43,282.44	$25,000.00	$18,282.44	$18,142.45	$139.99
Totals	$255,619.06		$106,936.33	$104,295.15	$2,641.18

Additionally, claims in this report will also show claims which were incurred received and processed timely by the contracted administrator but not applied to the appropriate filing for the Stoploss contracts of Specific and or Aggregate in the appropriate plan year. These claims will be shown in charts within this report and referred to the appropriate plan years. Details are provided in detail for each of the respective plan years 2014, 2013, 2012 and 2011.

Summary of Findings

First Level

The following chart shows the reimbursements not submitted by TPA 1 for **Specific Claims** as amounts are still due. 2014 information is illustrated based on significance of second level IRBNP.

Specific Stoploss

SUMMARY TOTALS JANUARY 2013 TO DECEMBER 31, 2013 SPECIFIC Stoploss ANALYSIS					
Name	Claims Pd	Spec Stoploss	Over Spec	Amount Reimb.	Amount Due Plan
5	$14,627.09	$20,000.00		$0.00	
1	$27,580.56	$25,000.00	$2,580.56	$2,580.56	$0.00
7	$38,672.52	$25,000.00	$13,672.52	$13,844.57	-$172.05
11	$47,378.95	$20,000.00	$27,378.95	$27,378.95	$0.00
12	$52,888.81	$20,000.00	$32,888.81	$32,888.81	$0.00
3	$58,092.36	$20,000.00	$38,092.36	$37,881.23	$211.13
Totals	$239,240.29		$114,613.20	$114,574.12	$39.08

SUMMARY TOTALS JANUARY 2012 TO DECEMBER 31, 2012 SPECIFIC Stoploss ANALYSIS					
Name	Claims Pd	Spec Stoploss	Over Spec	Amount Reimb.	Amount Due Plan
1	$31,536.24	$20,000.00	$11,536.24	$11,536.24	$0.00
7	$28,421.50	$25,000.00	$3,421.50	$3,421.50	$0.00
12	$94,514.15	$20,000.00	$74,514.15	$73,200.61	$1,313.54
3	$14,848.41	$20,000.00			
Totals	$169,320.30		$89,471.89	$88,158.35	$1,313.54

SUMMARY TOTALS JANUARY 2011 TO DECEMBER 31, 2011 SPECIFIC Stoploss ANALYSIS					
Name	Claims Pd	Spec Stoploss Deductible	Over Spec	Amount Reimb.	Amount Due Plan
1	$24,318.46	$17,500.00	$6,818.46	$6,781.13	$37.33
7	$20,250.23	$17,500.00	$2,750.23	$2,750.23	$0.00
WT	$60,916.94	$17,500.00	$43,416.94	$42,777.39	$639.55
Totals	$105,485.63		$52,985.63	$52,308.75	$676.88

Aggregate Stoploss

Plan Year	Aggregate Funding	Medical Claims	Rx Claims	Spec Reimbursement	Net Claims Subject to Aggregate	Aggregate Reimb calculated (-) = reimbursement to be paid by Stoploss (+) = Retention by Plan Sponsor	Aggregate Reimbursement Received	Total Due (-) to Plan Sponsor (+) to Stoploss
2014	$137,672.02	$215,981.96	$43,951.35	$104,295.15	$155,638.16	-$17,966.14	$0.00	-$17,966.14
2013	$166,187.34	$232,446.02	$68,988.70	$114,574.12	$186,860.60	-$20,673.26	$38,535.17	$17,861.91
2012	$145,264.68	$165,685.02	$53,231.80	$88,158.35	$130,758.47	$14,506.21	$0.00	
2011	$143,614.24	$144,941.67	$44,827.98	$52,308.75	$137,460.90	$6,153.34	$0.00	

In summary, the **first level** show from **Specific Stoploss** not received totals **$2,029.50** for Plan Years 2011, 2012 and 2013. The first level in regard to aggregate shows **$17,861.91** owed by Plan Sponsor to IAO Re based on Aggregate Reimbursement per Aggregate Accommodation provisions of Stoploss agreement.

Second Level

IRBNP (incurred received but not processed) are claims incurred and filed by the providers and received by the contracted administrator but not processed in a timely manner by the contracted administrator in the appropriate plan year for Stoploss contracts. These claims were extracted from the check registers submitted by TPA 1, (2011, 2012, 2013) and TPA 2 (2014).

Additionally, Contracted Administrators will process on the last day of the plan year to capture all claims and apply them to the respective specific Stoploss contracts and or aggregate Stoploss contracts. If this is not possible, the Contracted Administrator should contact the Stoploss Carrier and notify them of the claims and keep the contract open for these claims.

These claims are significant. The following will show the summary of the IRBNP claims applied to the specific years.

Aggregate claims are offset by the specific Stoploss reimbursements to show the outstanding aggregate retention, money retained by the plan sponsor (+) (Paducah Area Transit Health Plan) or Amounts to be received by the aggregate Stoploss (-).

Aggregate Stoploss

Aggregate Stoploss

Aggregate As Is	Aggregate Funding	Medical Claims	Rx Claims	Spec Reimbursement	Net Claims Subject to Aggregate	IRBNP	Aggregate Reimb calculated (-) = reimbursement to be paid by Stoploss (+) = Retention by Plan Sponsor	Aggregate Reimbursement Received	Total Due Plan Sponsor
Oct 24, 2014	$137,672.02	$215,981.96	$43,951.35	$104,295.15	$155,638.16		-$17,966.14	$0.00	-$17,966.14
Total Due Plan Sponsor									-$17,966.14
2013	$166,187.34	$232,446.02	$68,988.70	$114,574.12	$186,860.60	$33,273.14	-$53,946.40	$38,535.17	-$15,411.23
2012	$145,264.68	$165,685.02	$53,231.80	$88,158.35	$130,758.47	$1,394.15	$14,506.21	$0.00	
2011	$143,614.24	$144,941.67	$44,827.98	$52,308.75	$137,460.90	$2,934.40	$6,153.34	$0.00	
Total Plan Sponsor Owes 2011 to 2013 Underwriter									-$15,411.23

The IRBNP claims received in 2014 but should have been processed and applied to the 2013 plan year and Stoploss contracts totaled medical claims $28,888.64 and prescription claims $4,384.53 or a total of $33,273.17. These claims were not applied to the 2014 aggregate contract as they fell outside the 12/12 incurred and paid meaning incurred January 1, 2014 and paid by December 31, 2014. Reference: Data Analytics 2014 Plan Year for reference of detail. This is significant as the aggregate Stoploss for reimbursement should have been $53,946.40. The actual reimbursement received from TPA 1 filing was $38,535.17. This shows a total amount due to Plan Sponsor Health Plan of $15,411.23. From first level showing Plan Sponsor owed $17,861.91. Due to non process and application of these claims, TPA 1 is responsible for the $17,861.91 as well as $15,411.23 payable to Plan Sponsor. The total due is $33,273.14.

The IRBNP claims received in 2013 but should have been processed and applied to the 2012 plan year and Stoploss contracts totaled medical claims $1,394.15 and prescription claims $0 or a total of $1,394.15. These claims were not applied to the 2013 aggregate contract as they fell outside the 12/12 incurred and paid meaning incurred January 1, 2013 and paid by December 31, 2013. Reference: Data Analytics 2013 Plan Year for reference of detail. Nothing due Plan Sponsor.

The IRBNP claims received in 2012 but should have been processed and applied to the 2011 plan year and Stoploss contracts totaled medical claims $2,934.40 and prescription claims $0 or a total of $2,934.40. These claims were not applied to the 2012 aggregate contract as they fell outside the 12/12 incured and paid meaning incurred January 1, 2012 and paid by December 31, 2012. Reference: Data Analytics 2012 Plan Year for reference of detail. Nothing Due Plan Sponsor.

Specific Stoploss

The specific claims have been offset for each plan year for those claims considered IRBNP and added to the previous year for calculation of what the (+) or (-) is as it applies to the specific Stoploss.

SUMMARY TOTALS JANUARY 2014 TO DECEMBER 31, 2014 SPECIFIC Stoploss ANALYSIS

Name	Claims Pd	Spec Stoploss	Over Spec	Amount Reimb.	Amount Due Plan
5	$7,624.24	$25,000.00		$0.00	
1	$79,877.81	$35,000.00	$44,877.81	$74,296.62	-$29,418.81
7	$37,837.44	$40,000.00		$0.00	
11	$1,827.49	$40,000.00		$0.00	
12	$53,880.40	$40,000.00	$13,880.40	$11,856.08	$2,024.32
18	$43,282.44	$25,000.00	$18,282.44	$18,142.45	$139.99
Totals	$224,329.82		$77,040.65	$104,295.15	-$27,254.50

1 28,216.90 M, $1678.78 R = $29,895.68 IRBNP -$29,895.68 is subtracted from 2014 on claims paid and added to 2013 for proper application. 2014 $109,773.49 - $29,895.68 = $79,877.81. 2013 $27,580.56 + $29,895.68 = $57,476.24. **3** add 2013 $261.38 M, $47.79 R = $309.17 IRBNP to 2013 IRBNP $58,092.36 + $309.17 = $58,401.53. **7** subtract $1096.07 R IRBNP from 2014 add to 2013 $38,672.52 + $1,096.07 = $39,768.59. **11** subtract $297.49 R IRBNP from 2014 and add to 2013 $47,378.95 + $297.49 = $47,676.44

(**Reference**: *Data Analytics, 2014 Plan Year, IRBNP Extraction, Medical Claims, Prescription Claims*)

SUMMARY TOTALS JANUARY 2013 TO DECEMBER 31, 2013 SPECIFIC Stoploss ANALYSIS

Name	Claims Pd	Spec Stoploss	Over Spec	Amount Reimb.	Amount Due Plan
5	$14,627.09	$20,000.00		$0.00	
1	$57,312.51	$25,000.00	$32,312.51	$2,580.56	$29,731.95
7	$39,002.40	$25,000.00	$14,002.40	$13,844.57	$157.83
11	$47,676.44	$20,000.00	$27,676.44	$27,378.95	$297.49
12	$52,888.81	$20,000.00	$32,888.81	$32,888.81	$0.00
3	$58,401.53	$20,000.00	$38,401.53	$37,881.23	$520.30
Totals	$269,908.78		$145,281.69	$114,574.12	$30,707.57

7 subtract $766.16 M IRBNP from 2013 add to 2012 $28,421.50 + $766.16 = $29,187.66. **1** subtract $163.73 M IRBNP from 2013 add to

2012 $31,536.24 + $163.73 = $31,699.97. **12** add $408.50 M IRBNP to 2012 $94,514.15 + $408.50 = $94,922.65 (no subtraction for 12 as claims were not included for specific due to incurred out of date range of contract.

(***Reference***: *Data Analytics, 2013 Plan Year, IRBNP Extraction, Medical Claims, Prescription Claims*)

SUMMARY TOTALS JANUARY 2012 TO DECEMBER 31, 2012 SPECIFIC Stoploss ANALYSIS					
Name	Claims Pd	Spec Stoploss	Over Spec	Amount Reimb.	Amount Due Plan
1	$30,858.46	$20,000.00	$10,858.46	$11,536.24	-$677.78
7	$27,865.57	$25,000.00	$2,865.57	$3,421.50	-$555.93
12	$94,922.65	$20,000.00	$74,922.65	$73,200.61	$1,722.04
3	$14,848.41	$20,000.00			
Totals	$168,495.09		$88,646.68	$88,158.35	$488.33

1 subtract $841.51 M IRBNP from 2012 add to 2011 $24,318.46 + $841.51 = $25,159.97. **7** subtract $1,322.09 M IRBNP from 2012 add to 2011 $20,250.23 + $1,322.09 = $21,572.32.

(***Reference***: *Data Analytics, 2012 Plan Year, IRBNP Extraction, Medical Claims, Prescription Claims*)

SUMMARY TOTALS JANUARY 2011 TO DECEMBER 31, 2011 SPECIFIC Stoploss ANALYSIS					
Name	Claims Pd	Spec Stoploss Deductible	Over Spec	Amount Reimb.	Amount Due Plan
1	$25,159.97	$17,500.00	$7,659.97	$6,781.13	$878.84
7	$21,572.32	$17,500.00	$4,072.32	$2,750.23	$1,322.09
TW	$60,916.94	$17,500.00	$43,416.94	$42,777.39	$639.55
Totals	$107,649.23		$55,149.23	$52,308.75	$2,840.48

The following chart shows the specific claims which were incurred, processed and paid as to apply to the respective plan years. These amounts are extracted from the attached exhibits for each of the respective plan years.

Total Due Plan Sponsor - 2011 through 2013			
Specific	$6,781.88	To be paid to Plan Sponsor from TPA 1	
Aggregate	$15,411.23	To be paid to Plan Sponsor from TPA 1	
From TPA 1	$17,861.91	To be paid to Underwriter or Plan Sponsor due to IRBNP	
Total Due Plan Sponsor from TPA 1	$40,055.02		

Includes the calculated amounts due from the application of the IRBNP claims from 2011 through 2013. 2014 is a work in progress and the amounts due do not include the IRBNP for aggregate as there is none. But did include the claims as being subtracted out from 2014 Specific calculations. The calculations above are based on IRBNP being calculated appropriately based on plan year to which they should be applied.

Process

The process used and data received are based on the objective facts for each of the respective plan years.

Data Extraction

The information and data used are based on the check registers submitted by TPA 1 Plan Administrators (TPA) and TPA 2. Each of the respective plan years information was utilized. The data extraction process utilized is based initially on the check registers showing the date which the claim was incurred and the date the claim was paid. Once this information was compiled, a sort was done based on the incurred dates of the claims to get to what is know as IBNR. The IBNR was then extracted based on dates paid to view the probability of claims which fit the category of IRBNP.

From this extraction information for each of the respective plan years were sent to the Aggregator for additional analysis. United Claims Soultions was requested to incert information in specific categories with regard to these claims. The incertion categories provides objective data with regard to actual dates outside of the reported incurred and paid dates provided by TPA. This additional request of information included:

1. Co 1 Claim Number
2. Date Received by Co 1
3. Date Repriced by Co 1
4. Date EDI sent by Co 1
5. Co 1 File Name for EDI

This additional information provided the data for the true IRBNP claims vs IBNR claims. The following information provides dates from the Co 1 Claim Numbers by Co 1 as the dates received and the Co 1 File Name for EDI as the dates transmitted to TPA.

Co 1 Claim Number

Co 1 claim number shows the date the claim was received. The code used is: 120712C00374. The first two numbers shows the year (12 = 2012). The second two numbers shows the day of the month (07). The third two numbers shows the month (12 = December). Thus, this shows the claim was received by Co 1 on December 7, 2012.

Co 1 File Name

The Co 1 file name is also the EDI (Electronic Data Interface) which is the file prepared and transmitted to TPA. The code used is: TRD_PAR_111720121227837P.4010.edi.

1. TRD is the name of the TPA - TPA 1 Plan Administrators
2. PAR - shows the claim was a participating claim meaning in network with the PPO
3. The next eight digits shows the date the file was created and tranmitted. 11172012 which is 11-17-2012. This date shows the date the claim information was sent to the TPA for processing.

TPA Claim Number shows the date the claim was created by the TPA. The code for this claim number is:

TPA Claim Number

Claim Number: 212-035222-00
Per Joe xxxx - TPA 1 Plan Administrators: The only date information found in the claim number references the year the claim was incurred. The first 3 digits, 212, would indicate a service date in year 2012, 213 would indicate 2013, & so forth.

TPA 2 Claim Number

Unique medical claim number, formatted
YJJJSSSSSS
Y = Last digit of year entered
J = Julian date entered
S = Sequence number
Claim number: 268000077 = 2014 / 268 / = September 25

The codes on TPA and MAS show the dates the claim was processed. The comprison to the date received and processed provides the objective data for LAG, or the amount of time from the date the claim was recived to the date the claim was processed. This is imprtant as it will show if the TPA processed the claim in a timely manner.

(Subjective - TPA's or Contracted Administrators have an obligation to the plan to process expediantly at the end of the plan year to capture the claims for the current years Stoploss contract). Thus, all claims that can be processed that were received by the end of the current plan year are processed.

Additional analytics for the process shows the LAG or number of days for transmittal from the provider to date received and a second LAG for the number of days from receipt of claim to check date on the TPA. The LAG on TPA is improtant as it shows the number of days it took to process the claim received from Co 1 to the date the check was written.

Stoploss Contract

Specific

The specific Stoploss contract(s) have varing deductibles for individuals for each plan year. The specific Stoploss contract is a 15/12 incurred and paid. For claims to be eligible for the Stoploss contract they must be incurred October 1 and paid by December 31 in the following year.

Aggregate

The aggregate Stoploss contract is a 12/12 incurred and paid. For claims to be eligible for the Stoploss contract they must be incurred January 1 and paid by December 31 in the same year.

Claims are applied based on Stoploss contract. Specific claims are calculated and applied within the contract period. Claims in the Specific Stoploss are calculated based on the date the claim was incurred.

A claim incurred on October 2 in the previous plan year is applied to the specific deductible in relation to the participant specific deductible assigned. The claim incurred before January 1 in the current plan year is not applied to the aggregate Stoploss contract. The reimbursement received is applied to the current contract to reduce the aggregate in the current year. Claims incurred January 1 and and paid by December

31 in the current Stoploss contract are also allocated to the aggregate Stoploss contract in the current Stoploss contract year. Thus, these claims create the aggregate claims for the Stoploss contract.

Analysis

The analysis that follows is based on the objective facts (claims) in each of the respective Stoploss contract plan years. The initial findings are based on "AS Reported" by the TPA.

Information from the check registers for each plan year were reviewed for IBNR and then the IBNR was extracted to reveal the IRBNP claims for each of the respective plan years for application to view what the actual reimbursements for both specific Stoploss and aggregate Stoploss contracts would have been calculated if they had been processed by the TPA timely within the Stoploss contract plan years.

The following will show the information "As Reported" and with IRBNP applied. The results will validate based on fact the (+) or (-) for calculated reimbursements when the IRBNP is applied to the respective Stoploss contract years for Specific and Aggregate calculations. All data received was from TPA 1 Plan Administrators and or TPA 2, Contracted Administrators), for the calculations. Additional information for validation in date of claims received and transmitted to the Contracted Administrators was received from (Aggregator) to substantiate the IRBNP claims for application.

Each of the respective plan years calculations are applied and detailed in the following calculations. The structure for this analysis are plan years 2014, 2013, 2012 and 2011.

Data Analytics

2014 Plan Year

IRNBP Extraction

Medical Claims

The claims extracted are from the check registers submitted by TPA 2 but incurred while TPA 1 Plan Administrators was the administrator for claims in plan year 2013.

CHKNO	FROMDT	Date Received by Co 1	Co 1 Claim #	Date Repriced by Co 1	Date EDI Sent by Co 1	CHKDT	AMT	PAYEE	LASTNAME	
417	12/11/13	12/23/13	131223C1548	12/24/13	12/25/13	1/31/14	$438.58	LOURDES HOSPITAL	1	
375	12/13/13	12/24/13	131224C3181	12/27/13	12/28/13	1/31/14	$13,120.41	JACKSON PURCHASE MEDICAL ASSOC	1	
472	11/22/13	12/17/13	131217C1044	12/30/13	12/31/13	3/7/14	$13,286.48	JACKSON PURCHASE MEDICAL ASSOC	1	
486	12/17/13	12/27/13	131227C1913	12/30/13	12/31/13	3/21/14	$1,313.63	ORTHOPEDIC INSTITUTE OF W KY	1	
385	12/18/13	12/27/13	131227C1914	12/30/13	12/31/13	1/31/14	$57.80	TOTAL LIFE CARE PLLC	1	$28,216.90
388	12/26/13	12/23/13	131223C1547	12/24/13	12/25/13	1/31/14	$58.64	JAMES K TURNBO MD	2	
402	12/2/13	12/17/13	131217C1046	12/30/13	12/31/13	1/31/14	$121.72	BAPTIST HEALTH OF PADUCAH	2	$180.36
397	11/8/13	12/24/13	131224C2824	12/30/13	12/31/13	1/31/14	$97.74	FOUR RIVERS INTERNAL MEDICINE PLLC	3	
399	11/13/13	12/24/13	131224C2825	12/30/13	12/31/13	1/31/14	$105.00	FOUR RIVERS INTERNAL MEDICINE PLLC	3	
387	12/2/13	12/24/13	131224C2823 - IF TIN 611367882 IS CORRECT	12/30/13	12/31/13	1/31/14	$58.64	FOUR RIVERS INTERNAL MEDICINE PLLC	3	$261.38
411	12/31/13	12/24/13	131224C2826	12/30/13	12/31/13	1/31/14	$230.00	PURCHASE DERM ENT PLLC	4	$230.00
							$28,888.64			

These IRBNP claims should have been processed in the 2013 Plan Year. File would have been received by TPA 1 and could have been processed with checks written to meet the specific and aggregate requirements in 2013.

Prescription Claims

The claims extracted are from the check registers submitted by TPA 2 but incurred while TPA 1 Plan Administrators was the administrator for claims in plan year 2013. These claims should have been processed in the 2013 Plan Year as they would have bee received by TPA 1 in the 2013 Plan Year.

CHKNO	CLMNO	CHKDT	FROMDT	AMT	PAYEE	LASTNAME
383	21000258	1/31/14	12/3/13	$47.79	HEALTHSMART RX, INC.	3
426	21000234	1/31/14	12/3/13	$1,678.87	HEALTHSMART RX, INC.	1
381	21000222	1/31/14	12/4/13	$30.37	HEALTHSMART RX, INC.	5
420	21000229	1/31/14	12/4/13	$562.56	HEALTHSMART RX, INC.	6
424	21000245	1/31/14	12/4/13	$1,096.07	HEALTHSMART RX, INC.	7
407	21000230	1/31/14	12/6/13	$167.91	HEALTHSMART RX, INC.	8
416	21000231	1/31/14	12/9/13	$329.74	HEALTHSMART RX, INC.	9
406	21000257	1/31/14	12/10/13	$149.04	HEALTHSMART RX, INC.	10
379	21000259	1/31/14	12/13/13	$24.69	HEALTHSMART RX, INC.	4
415	21000256	1/31/14	12/13/13	$297.49	HEALTHSMART RX, INC.	11
		Year-to-Date Total:		$4,384.53		

The amount of $4,384.53 should have been processed in the 2013 Plan Year. This would have been for both the Specific and Aggregate Stoploss Contracts for the 2013 Plan Year.

Summary 2014

The following claims should have been included in the 2013 Plan Year and applied to the Specific and Aggregate.

Category	Medical Claims	Rx Claims	Total
IRBNP for 2013 Application	$28,888.64	$4,384.53	$33,273.17

2013 Plan Year

IRNBP Extraction

Medical Claims

DATE Paid	DATE INCURRED	Date Received by Co 1	Co 1 claim #	Date Repriced by Co 1	Date EDI Sent by Co 1	Co 1 file name	CLAIM NUMBER	INSURED / PATIENT NAME	PAYEE NAME	AMOUNT
9/13/13	1/24/12	7/12/12	1207712C00374	8/15/12	no claim history	no claim history	212-002094-03	15	WESTERN BAPTIST HOSPI	-$35.20
9/13/13	1/24/12	7/12/12	1207712C00374	8/15/12	no claim history	no claim history	212-002094-04	15	WESTERN BAPTIST HOSPI	$35.20
1/15/13	7/18/12	11/16/12	121116C0554	11/16/12	11/17/12	TRD_PAR_1117201212278371P.4010.edi	212-035221-00	12	PURCHASE CANCER GROUP	$370.25
1/15/13	7/18/12	11/16/12	121116C0553	11/16/12	11/17/12	TRD_PAR_1117201212278371P.4010.edi	212-035222-00	12	PURCHASE CANCER GROUP	$38.25
9/13/13	8/3/12	8/21/12	120821C0791	8/21/12	8/22/12	TRD_PAR_0822201209058371.4010.edi	212-021934-01	4	WESTERN BAPTIST HOSPI	-$28.56
9/13/13	8/3/12	8/21/12	120821C0791	8/21/12	8/22/12	TRD_PAR_0822201209058371.4010.edi	212-021934-02	4	WESTERN BAPTIST HOSPI	$28.56
3/19/13	9/11/12	10/2/12	121002C1481	10/2/12	10/3/12	TRD_PAR_1003201207078371P.4010.edi	212-037887-00	1	ORTHOPEDIC INSTITUTE	$163.73
1/15/13	10/31/12	11/16/12	121116C0547	11/16/12	11/17/12	TRD_PAR_1117201212278371P.4010.edi	212-035167-00	7	PADUCAH MAGNETIC RESO	$655.59
1/15/13	10/31/12	11/16/12	121116C0546	11/16/12	11/17/12	TRD_PAR_1117201212278371P.4010.edi	212-035230-00	7	RADIOLOGY GROUP OF PA	$110.57
1/31/13	12/5/12	12/28/12	121228C0055	12/28/12	12/29/12	TRD_PAR_1229201212028371P.4010.edi	212-036669-00	4	TOTAL LIFE CARE PLLC	$55.76
										$1,394.15

Summary 2013

Category	Medical Claims	Rx Claims	Total
IRBNP for 2012 Application	$1,394.15	$0.00	$1,394.15

2012 Plan Year

IRNBP Extraction

Medical Claims

CHECK / TRANS #	DATE PAID	DATE INCURRED	Co 1 Date Received	Co 1 claim #	Co 1 Date Repriced	INSURED / PATIENT NAME	PAYEE NAME	Payment Amount
503	1/16/12	12/2/11	12/27/11	111227C00714	12/27/11	4	DAVID S CHALKE DC	$15.00
545	3/30/12	1/24/11	2/2/11	110202C00482	2/2/11	6	OPHTHALMOLOGY GROUP L	$83.00
519	2/15/12	11/1/11	11/15/11	111115C00142	11/15/11	13	TOTAL LIFE CARE PLLC	$75.00
686	8/31/12	6/30/11	9/13/11	110913C00332	9/13/11	14	DAVID A MEYER MD	$54.40
492	1/16/12	12/19/11	12/30/11	111230C00125	12/30/11	14	COMPREHENSIVE NEUROLO	$58.64
536	3/15/12	12/28/10	1/7/11	110107C00236	1/17/11	10	W KENTUCKY SURGICAL A	$92.80
497	1/16/12	9/29/11	12/27/11	111227C00717	12/27/11	10	LOURDES PHYSICIAN SER	$36.00
499	1/16/12	12/12/11	12/27/11	111227C00396	12/27/11	7	LOURDES HOSPITAL	$1,322.09
566	4/13/12	6/3/11	7/21/11	110721C00486	7/21/11	17	JACKSON PURCHASE MEDI	$105.92
500	1/16/12	12/12/11	12/12/11	111227C00716	12/27/11	17	LINCARE INC	$65.42
515	1/31/12	11/30/11	12/12/11	111212C00329	12/12/11	3	COMPREHENSIVE PREMIER	$105.92
497	1/16/12	12/2/11	12/27/11	111227C00715	12/27/11	1	LOURDES PHYSICIAN SER	$105.92
496	1/16/12	12/6/11	12/27/11	111227C00374	12/27/11	1	RADIOLOGY GROUP OF PA	$24.11
497	1/16/12	12/7/11	12/27/11	111227C00713	12/27/11	1	LOURDES PHYSICIAN SER	$615.57
495	1/16/12	12/6/11	12/28/11	111228C00282	12/28/11	1	RACHEL A CROWLEY PA-C	$20.91
510	1/31/12	11/2/11	12/27/11 12/27/11 11/18/11	111227C00192 OR 111227C00191 OR 111118C00123	12/27/11 12/27/11 11/18/11	1	TOTAL LIFE CARE PLLC	$75.00
518	1/31/12	10/21/11	12/8/11	111208C00702	12/8/11	16	JACKSON PURCHASE MEDI	$78.70
								$2,934.40

Summary 2012

Category	Medical Claims	Rx Claims	Total
IRBNP for 2011 Application	$2,934.40	$0.00	**$2,934.40**

Aggregate Stoploss

Aggregate As Is	Aggregate Funding	Medical Claims	Rx Claims	Spec Reimbursement	Net Claims Subject to Aggregate	IRBNP	Aggregate Reimb calculated (-) = reimbursement to be paid by Stoploss (+) = Retention by Plan Sponsor	Aggregate Reimbursement Received	Total Due Plan Sponsor
Sept 30, 2014	$124,733.17	$207,589.47	$34,653.07	$86,152.70	$156,089.84		-$31,356.67	$0.00	-$31,356.67
Total Due Plan Sponsor									-$31,356.67
2013	$166,187.34	$232,446.02	$68,988.70	$114,574.12	$186,860.60	$33,273.14	-$53,946.40	$38,535.17	-$15,411.23
2012	$145,264.68	$165,685.02	$53,231.80	$88,158.35	$130,758.47	$2,251.27	$14,506.21	$0.00	
2011	$143,614.24	$144,941.67	$44,827.98	$52,308.75	$137,460.90	$2,934.40	$6,153.34	$0.00	
Total Plan Sponsor Owes 2011 to 2013 Underwriter									-$15,411.23

The amount calculated shows Plan Sponsor is due (-) and Plan Sponsor owes (+).

Applying the data for IRBNP in the amount of $33,273.14 processed in the 2014 Plan Year as an IBNR can not be applied to the Aggregate Stoploss for the 2014 Plan Year based on the dates the claim was incurred. This amount became a 100% cost to Plan Sponsor in the 2014 Plan Year. The amounts received in Specific Stoploss reimbursements off set the net claims subject to aggregate in each the respective 2014, 2013, 2012 and 2013 Plan Years. These amounts were left unmodified as an offset for claims subject to Aggregate. With the amount $33,273.14 not eligible for aggregate Stoploss in the 2014 Plan Year provided the amount Plan Sponsor would owe to Underwriter for Aggregate Accommodation is $17,861.91.

With the IBNR for 2013 extracted for IRNBP is applied to the 2013 in the amount of $33,273.14. With this calculation, TPA 1 Plan Administrators is responsible for paying the $17,861.91 to Underwriter and $15,411.23 to Plan Sponsor as the combination of these would have resulted in application to the Aggregate Stoploss Contract for 2013.

Exhibit A

Administration Agreement

TPA 1 Plan Administrators, Inc

For

Plan Sponsor

Agreement important provisions

The administrative agreement was effective as of January 1, 2010 for a period of 36 months. (Page 1)

III. Duties of TPA 1

3.2.1.10 Use its best efforts in the normal course of its services hereunder to identify claims that may be subject to reimbursement, based upon the existence of any Stoploss or Reinsurance Policy. In no event will TPA 1 be heald liable for any claims no covered or not paid by the Stoploss or Reinsurance Carrier.
3.3.3 Maintain reinsurance reporting.
3.7.2 Report of aggregate claims paid (monthly).
3.7.3 Reports of claims incurred and reported but not paid, also known as a pended claims report (annually).

V. General Provisions

5.6 Assignment. Neither Party shall, without the consent of the other in advance and in writing, assign or transfer any right, benefit, obligation or duty under the terms of theis Agreement.

VI. Term of Agreement

6.1 Term. This Agreement shall commence on January 1, 2010 and shall continue in effect until expiration, unless terminated as provided for below. This Agreement will automatically renew for additional two (2) year terms unless notice is received given by either party of non renewal 90 days or more prior to expiration.
6.2.2 By Default. Should either party default in the performance of any of the terms or conditions of this Agreement, the other party may deliver written notice (personally or by Certified mail) to the defaulting party thereof specifying the matters in default.

TPA 1

Third Party Administration Agreement

Rev 0809

Third Party Administration Agreement

THIS AGREEMENT is made by and between Plan Sponsor, hereinafter referred to as the **Plan Sponsor**, whose principal address is xxxx, and TPA 1 Plan Administrators, hereinafter referred to as **TPA 1**, whose principal address is xxxxx with respect to the Benefit Plan issued by the Plan Sponsor to the eligible covered employees and dependents. This Agreement is to be in effect as of January 1, 2010 and shall continue for a period of 36 Months..

WHEREAS, the Plan Sponsor has established a self funded employee welfare benefit plan pursuant to the Employee Retirement Income Security Act of 1974, as amended, (the "Plan") for certain employees of the Plan Sponsor and for certain dependents of such employees ("Participants"); and

WHEREAS, TPA 1 is in the business of providing administrative services in conjunction with such Plans, and the Plan Sponsor desires to engage TPA 1 to perform the services enumerated herein below:

NOW, THEREFORE, in consideration of the premises and of the mutual promises and covenants contained herein, the parties agree as follows:

I. PLAN

1.1 Plan Document. All services to be provided by TPA 1 hereunder shall be performed pursuant to the provisions of the Plan Document, as amended. A copy of the Plan Document and any amendments thereto shall be deemed to form part of this Agreement for such purpose.

1.2 Interpretation of the Plan. The Plan Sponsor shall be the sole and final arbiter as to the interpretation of the Plan and as to the payment of benefits hereunder. TPA 1 shall consult with the Plan Sponsor in the event extraordinary benefit matters arise. In the event an exception is to be made, the Plan Sponsor will notify TPA 1 in writing of such exception.

II. SCOPE OF RELATIONSHIP

2.1 Agency. In performing the services hereunder, TPA 1 is acting solely as the agent of the Plan Sponsor, and the respective rights of the parties shall be determined in accordance with the laws of agency. In the event that the Plan Sponsor fails to comply with any federal or state law, TPA 1 shall not be liable in any action brought with regard to such failure.

2.2 Fiduciary. TPA 1 is not and shall not be deemed to be a fiduciary of the Plan. Nor shall TPA 1 be considered to be the "Plan Administrator" for purposes of ERISA. Rather, the duties of TPA 1 hereunder are ministerial in nature; and this Agreement shall not be deemed to confer or delegate to TPA 1 any discretionary authority or discretionary responsibility in the administration of the Plan.

2.3 Communications. TPA 1 shall be entitled to rely, without questions, upon any written or oral communication from the Person designated by the Plan Sponsor. Until amended by letter, the following individuals shall be so authorized: Chuck 4, Trustee and Kim Adair, Trustee.

2.4 **Parties.** This Agreement is between TPA 1 and the Plan Sponsor, and does not create any rights or legal relationships between TPA 1 and any of the Participants or Beneficiaries under the Plan.

III. DUTIES OF TPA 1

3.1 **Documentation.** TPA 1 shall review the existing Plan Document, and assist in the review of the Plan Booklets (describing the benefits of the plan). The Plan Sponsor understands that ERISA requires that its employee welfare benefit plan be established and maintained pursuant to a written instrument (plan instrument or trust instrument); and the Plan Sponsor agrees that TPA 1 shall have no responsibility with respect to such instrument or with respect to the preparation or validity of such instrument.

3.2 **Claims Services.** TPA 1 agrees to perform the below-enumerated services with respect to the processing and payment of claims under the Plan:

    3.2.1 **Services.** TPA 1 agrees to:

        3.2.1.1 Provide claim forms to the Plan Sponsor for submitting claims to TPA 1;

        3.2.1.2 Receive claims and claims documentation;

        3.2.1.3 Correspond with the Participants and Providers of service if additional information is deemed by TPA 1 to be necessary to complete the processing of claims;

        3.2.1.4 Coordinate benefits payable under the Plan with other benefit plans, if any;

3.2.1.5   Determine the amount of benefits payable under the Plan;

3.2.1.6   Prepare disbursement checks for the amount of benefits determined to be payable under the Plan;

3.2.1.7   Provide customer service personnel between the hours of 8:00 a.m. and 5:00 p.m. Mountain Standard Time, Mondays through Fridays, except holidays; unless other specific times have been agreed upon.

3.2.1.8   Provide notice to Participants as to the reason(s) for denial of benefits and provide for the review of denied claims; provided, however, that such review shall be advisory to the Plan Sponsor in accordance with Section 1.2 above and shall not be deemed to be an exercise of discretion by TPA 1 in accordance with Section 2.2 above;

3.2.1.9   Use its best efforts in the normal course of its services hereunder to identify claims for which there is the potential for collection of amounts paid to, or on behalf of, Participants through subrogation of rights of Participants and to notify the Plan Sponsor of such claims;

3.2.1.10 Use its best efforts in the normal course of its services hereunder to identify claims that may be subject to reimbursement, based upon the existence of any Stoploss or Reinsurance Policy. In no event will TPA 1 be held liable

3.2.1.11   TPA 1 will also forward payment of Plan Sponsor agreed upon disbursements to all contracted insurance carriers, brokers, agents, consultants the third party administrator (TPA 1) and other third party suppliers to the Plan.

3.2.1.12   Under no circumstances whatsoever will TPA 1 release any disbursements or Plan payments prior to receiving confirmation of good funds on deposit in the Plan's bank accounts sufficient to cover the amount of the disbursements to be released.

3.3 Administrative Services. TPA 1 agrees to:

3.3.1   Maintain member enrollment for eligibility for payment of claims and census data;

3.3.2   Provide accounting details of all billing and collections;

3.3.3   Maintain reinsurance reporting;

3.3.4   Provide experience reporting for coverages;

3.3.5   Provide enrollment forms and in conjunction with the PBM provide identification cards to the Plan Sponsor for distribution to Plan participants.

3.4 Practices and Procedures. In performing such services, TPA 1 shall employ its standard practices and procedures, whether written or otherwise; provided, however, such performance shall be subject to the provision of this Agreement, including, but not limited to Section 1.2.

[Continued from previous page:] for any claims not covered or not paid by the Stoploss or Reinsurance Carrier.

3.5 **Recovery of Payment.** In the event payment is made to or on behalf of an ineligible employee, Participant or any ineligible dependent of an employee Participant or that a payment is made in excess of the amount properly payable, TPA 1 shall:make two demands with respect to the Participant/Provider in writing for the return of such payment or overpayment and report the result of such effort to the Plan Sponsor. TPA 1 shall have no further obligation with respect to any such payment or overpayment, except that TPA 1 is hereby authorized to offset any such overpayment against any unpaid claim of such employee, Participant or any dependent thereof unless advised otherwise by the Plan Sponsor.

3.6 **Records and Files.** TPA 1 shall establish and maintain a record keeping system concerning the services to be performed hereunder. All such records shall be the property of the Plan Sponsor and shall be delivered to the Plan Sponsor upon termination of this Agreement, at his cost, subject to the right of TPA 1 to copy and retain all or any of such records as it deems in its best interest to do so. All such records shall be available for inspection by the Plan Sponsor at any time during normal business hours at the offices of TPA 1 in Phoenix, Arizona, upon reasonable prior notice.

3.7 **Reports.** TPA 1 shall provide the following to the Plan Sponsor:

    3.7.1   Claims Check registers (weekly or bi-monthly);

    3.7.2   Report of aggregate claims paid (monthly);

    3.7.3   Reports of claims incurred and reported but not paid, also known as a pended claims report (annually);

    3.7.4   Any other reports mutually agreed upon.

3.8 **Confidentiality of Personal Information.** TPA 1 shall take all reasonable precautions to prevent disclosure or use of the information for a purpose unrelated to administration of the plan, except in the following instances:

- 3.8.1 In response to a court order;

- 3.8.2 For an examination conducted by the Commissioner of Insurance;

- 3.8.3 For an audit or investigation conducted under the Employee Retirement Income Security Act of 1974 (29 U.S.C. 1001, et seq.);

- 3.8.4 To or at the request of the insurer or Plan Sponsor; or

- 3.8.5 With the written consent of the identified individual or his or her legal representative.

3.9 **Limitation of Liability** – Under ERISA, the Corporation (TPA 1) shall be considered the Plan supervisor, but the Corporation shall not be liable for any loss to the Employer (the Plan Sponsor) resulting from the performance of the Corporation's duties hereunder, except for losses resulting directly from the fraudulent or criminal acts of the agents or employees of the Corporation, whether acting alone or in concert with others; except that if such act or acts shall have been performed in concert with an agent or employee of the Employer. The Employer shall bear liability for the resulting loss. Further, all governmental reporting requirements are the sole responsibility of the Employer.

IV. DUTIES OF PLAN SPONSOR

4.1 **Account.** The Plan Sponsor shall establish, maintain and fund a checking account(s) ("Account") for the payment of benefits and expenses under the Plan. The Plan Sponsor shall be liable for all checks issued against the Account. TPA 1 shall provide Plan Sponsor with a report or tape for reconciliation.

4.2 **Service Fee.** The Plan Sponsor agrees to pay TPA 1 a Service Fee as illustrated in Exhibit A based on the number of active Participants covered under the Plan at the beginning of each calendar month. The Plan Sponsor agrees to pay the Service Fee, and all other fees as determined in this Section, on or before the 10th of each calendar month for which services are being rendered. "COBRA" participants are considered active participants for purposes of calculating the Service Fee.

4.3 **Substantial Change.** Any substantial change in the Plan or services requested by the Plan Sponsor, which requires additional programs, processes or personnel, may require an adjustment of service fees which will be mutually agreed upon in writing prior to to the implementation of such changes or additional services.

4.4 **Audit fees.** TPA 1 recognizes that from time to time the Plan Sponsor may wish to perform (or have performed) an audit for financial statement purposes, performance standard related, claims payment or other purposes. The Plan Sponsor agrees to pay TPA 1 on an hourly rate for the staff time involved in such audit as shown in Schedule A.

4.5 **Other Fees and Expenses.** The Plan Sponsor shall be responsible for paying promptly all other contracted fees, services, and insurance premiums.

4.6 **Taxes and Other Assessments.** The Plan Sponsor will pay TPA 1 within a reasonable time after assessment, any tax or charge assessed against TPA 1 which may be incurred by reason of (a) a ruling or other determination by an Insurance Department or other governmental authority, to the effect that any fees or charges payable under Section 4.2 or the amount of claim payments made in accordance with the Plan and Section III of this Agreement, is an insurance premium and subject to the premium tax provisions of the applicable statutes, including any retroactive assessment;

(b) a change in any charges imposed on TPA 1 by any public body, exclusive of Federal or State Income Taxes, which affect this Agreement.

    4.6.1 Tax Collection. The Plan Sponsor will promptly pay to TPA 1 all state and local taxes which may be imposed on the Plan Sponsor or TPA 1 as a result of this Agreement. TPA 1 agrees to remit these to the proper authorities in a timely fashion.

    4.6.2 Tax Liability. It is agreed that nothing in this Agreement will be deemed to confer on TPA 1 any responsibility for any federal, state or local tax liability which may be imposed upon TPA 1, the Plan Sponsor, trust, Administration, Fiduciary or any Participant or Beneficiary of the Plan.

    4.6.3 Government Reporting. The Plan Sponsor shall bear sole responsibility and liability for all governmental reporting requirements for the Plan and the Plan Sponsor, even if TPA 1 is contracted to prepare or advise on the preparation of any such reports.

4.7 Census. The Plan Sponsor agrees to furnish TPA 1 such information as may be necessary or required by TPA 1 from time to time to maintain adequate eligibility records of Plan Sponsor's Participants.

4.8 Liability for Benefits. It is understood and agreed that liability for payment of benefits under the Plan is the liability of the Employer and that TPA 1 shall not have any duty to use any of its funds for the payment of such benefits. Both parties recognize that this specifically includes Medicare Secondary Payer Claims, even though such claims may not be specifically allowed by Plan language or may be time-barred under the terms of the Plan Document.

4.9 **Indemnification.** The Plan Sponsor agrees to protect, to indemnify and to hold harmless TPA 1 from any and all actions causes of actions, suits, claims, judgments, settlements, liabilities, damages penalties, losses, and/or expenses including without limitation, extra contract damages, court costs, attorneys' fees, any punitive or exemplary damages, resulting from or arising out of or in connection with, any acts or omissions of TPA 1 under this agreement, unless it is determined that the liability therefore was the direct and sole consequence of willful misconduct, criminal negligence or criminal fraud on the part of TPA 1, its officers, directors, or employees, in the performance of their duties under this Agreement.

V. GENERAL PROVISIONS

5.1 **Entire Contract.** This Agreement, together with any Exhibits, Attachments and Amendments appended hereto, constitutes the entire Agreement between the parties. No representation, understanding or agreements that are not expressly contained herein shall be binding or enforceable. No modification of the terms or provisions of this Agreement shall be effective unless evidenced by written amendment hereto, signed by an authorized officer of both the Plan Sponsor and of TPA 1.

5.2 **Applicable Law.** This Agreement shall be deemed to have been made and entered into in the State of Arizona, and shall be construed and enforced according to the laws of the State of Arizona.

5.3 **Arbitration.** If any dispute shall arise between the Plan Sponsor and TPA 1, either before or after termination of this Agreement, with reference to the interpretation of this Agreement or the rights of either party with respect to any transaction under this Agreement, the dispute shall be referred to three arbitrators, one to be chosen by each party and the third by the two so chosen. If either party refuses or neglects to appoint an arbitrator within thirty (30) days after the receipt of written notice from the other party requesting it to do so, the requesting party may nominate two arbitrators who shall choose the third. In the event, the two arbitrators do not agree on the selection of the third arbitrator within (30) days after both arbitrators have been named, then the third arbitrator shall be selected pursuant to the commercial arbitration rules of the American Arbitration Association. The arbitrators shall consider this Agreement an honorable engagement rather than merely a legal obligation; they are relieved of all judicial formalities and may abstain from following the strict rules of law. The decision of a majority of the arbitrators shall be final and binding on both the Plan Sponsor and TPA 1, and judgment upon the award rendered by the arbitrators may be entered into any court having jurisdiction thereof. The expense of the arbitrators and of the arbitration shall be equally divided between the Plan Sponsor and TPA 1. Arbitration is the sole remedy for disputes arising under this Agreement.

5.4 **Waiver.** Failure of either party at anytime to require performance by the other party of any provision of this Agreement shall not be deemed to be a continuing waiver of that provision or a waiver of any other provision of this Agreement.

5.5 **Notices.** All notices provided for herein shall be deemed to have been given or made when deposited, with proper postage affixed, into the United States mail and addressed to the other party at their respective address set forth above or such other addresses as any of the parties hereto may designate in writing to the other from time to time for such purposes.

5.6 **Assignment.** Neither Party shall, without the consent of the other in advance and in writing, assign or transfer any right, benefit, obligation or duty under the terms of this Agreement.

5.7 **Amendments.** This agreement or any part thereof may be modified at any time by the mutual agreement of the parties, but such modification or amendment must be in writing.

VI. TERM OF AGREEMENT

6.1 **Term.** This Agreement shall commence on January 1, 2010 and shall continue in effect until expiration, unless terminated as provided for below. This Agreement will automatically renew for additional two (2) year terms unless notice is received given by either party of non renewal 90 days or more prior to expiration.

6.2 **Termination By Notice.** After this Agreement has been in effect for twelve (12) months, either Party may terminate this Agreement for any reason at any time by providing written notice to the other party. The notice shall specify any effective date of termination which shall be not less than ninety (90) days nor more than one hundred eighty (180) days after the date of receipt of the notice by the other party. If the notice does not specify a date of termination, the effective date of termination shall be ninety (90) days after receipt of the notice by the other party. In the event of termination by the Plan Sponsor, or any successor thereof, for any reason other than By Default or By Law TPA 1 will be due twelve (12) months administration fees at the then prevailing rate based on the census at the date of termination.

    6.2.2 **By Default.** Should either party default in the performance of any of the terms or conditions of this Agreement, the other party may deliver written notice (personally or by certified mail) to the defaulting party thereof specifying the matters in default. The defaulting party shall have thirty (30) calendar days after its receipt of the written notice to either cure or refute such default. If the defaulting party fails to cure or refute the default within such period, this Agreement may be terminated at any time thereafter, prior to the default being subsequently cured, by delivery upon the breaching party (personally or by certified mail) of a written thirty (30) day termination notice.

    6.2.3 **By Law.** If any state or federal law or regulation is enacted or promulgated which prohibits the performance of any of the duties hereunder, or if any law is interpreted to prohibit such performance, this Agreement shall automatically terminate as of the effective date of such prohibition.

6.3 **Effect of Termination.** As of the effective date of termination of this Agreement, TPA 1 shall have no further duties of performance hereunder, other than Run Out Claims Processing as described in Section 6.3.1 below. This period between notice of termination and the effective date of termination shall be used to effect an orderly transfer of records and funds, if any, from TPA 1 to the Plan Sponsor or to such person as the Plan Sponsor may designate in writing. Any records transfer shall be completed within thirty (30) calendar days of the termination date.

    6.3.1 **Run-out Claims.** In the event of termination of this agreement, TPA 1 will process claims incurred prior to the termination date for three (3) months after the termination date, at the rate of one hundred and twenty five per cent (125%) of the Service Fee in effect on the termination date. Claims received after three (3) months will be processed by TPA 1 at $20.00 per claim. All duties of the Plan Sponsor shall remain in effect for a period ending thirty days following cessation of all claims payment by TPA 1.

VII. ATTACHMENTS TO THIS AGREEMENT

7.1 Any schedules attached to this agreement will be considered an integral part of this agreement.

IN WITNESS WHEREOF, the parties have executed this Agreement as of the effective date first appearing above.

PLAN SPONSOR: TPA 1 PLAN ADMINISTRATORS

BY:_____ BY:
Company Representative   Company Representative
Title: **Human Resources, Dir.**   Title: **CEO**
Dated: **12-8-09**   Dated: **12-3-09**

SCHEDULE A
FEE SCHEDULE

THIS SCHEDULE is attached to and made a part of the Third Party Administration Agreement by and between the Plan Sponsor and TPA 1 and sets forth fees for the Plan Year as follows:

Medical Administration	$ 19.00 PEPM
COBRA and HIPAA Administration	$ 1.00 PEPM
Fee per RX script Filled	$ .50
Online claims viewing	Included
Set Up Fee	Waived

Exhibit B

Stoploss Agreement

Underwriter

For

Plan Sponsor

Plan Years 2014 and 2013

Agreement important provisions

Contract Period: January 1 to December 31 of each of the respective plan years 2014 and 2013.

Specific Stoploss: Includes Specific Advance. 2014 contract basis: 15/12. Specific Deductible: $25,000. 2013 contract basis: 15/12. Specific Deductible: $20,000.

Specific Limitations 2014:

7	$40,000
1	$35,000
11	$40,000
12	$40,000

Specific Limitations 2013:

7	$25,000
1	$25,000

Aggregate Stoploss: Includes Aggregate Advancement. 2014 contract basis: 12/12. 2013 contract basis 12/12.

NOTE: *A significance in the specific limitations on the individuals above in the calculation of the specific reibursments to be received per plan year. With the individuals above, and IRBNP not processed created additional reibursements for each of the respective individuals and plan years due to increases above the scheduled Stoploss dedcutibles. Non process of claims in the respective plan years created additional liability to TPA 1 for non processing of claims received and considered IRBNP.*

Based on the objective facts provided for analysis, the following chart shows the findings.

I reserve the right to change, modify or correct any and all comments or conclusions expressed in my written observations should I be given additional information that would warrant such actions.

Respectfully Submitted,

F. Randall Childers, Jr., CFC, DABFE
Certified Forensic Consultant
Diplomate American Board of Forensic Examiners

Pharmacy Agreements Analysis

The following is a case where the retail pharmacy was having issues with how the structure of the contracts with the computer company, PSAO organization, suppliers, PBM's and others as it related to their revenue. The following is a summarized evaluation regarding the findings of current agreements, contracts, pricing and current methods used from vendors for payment of billings. This was basically done in two levels 1. Agreements and 2. Data, Computer import of pricing and quantity of inventory, (inventory cost, retail pricing and profit margins).

OVERVIEW

OBJECTIVE

Evaluation of current methods, pricing, review the potential for reducing losses and increasing profits from Anywhere Pharmacy use of Computer Company Rx, AB Drug Corporation, Consulting Organization with Analysis of Agreements / Contracts and Data Supplied.

The report is broken out in two sections.

1. Agreements and Contracts
2. Data Analytics

RESERVE

We reserve the right to change, modify or correct any and all comments or conclusions expressed in the written observations should we be given additional information that would warrant such actions.

INFORMATION REQUEST

The following information was requested for analysis and review.

AGREEMENTS / CONTRACTS

> Contract with AB,
> Contract with Computer CompanyRx pharmacy software.
> Contracts with PBM's
> Contracts with PSAO (Pharmacy Services Administrative Organization)
> Medicare Pricing Agreements
> Medicaid Pricing Agreements

DATA

> System Data via Computer CompanyRx pharmacy software in excel compatible format.
> Copies of invoices from AB or in excel l compatible format.
> Copies of Billings from and Payments to PBM's, Insurance Companies, PSAO, Medicare and Medicaid or in excel compatible format.
> Copy of Inventory last completed and back to inception with Computer CompanyRx pharmacy software or in excel compatible format.

Review of Agreements Contracts

Each of the different agreements / contracts were reviewed and an analysis of each was done for content, completeness, providing any and all details described, full disclosure of any and all fees associated and detail of cost structures with DIR / Clawback provisions specific to the PSAO and PBM Agreements. The analysis of this information would provide the TRANSPARENCY of the agreements executed by Anywhere Pharmacy.

CPA MASTER PROGRAM AGREEMENT

Requests

After review of the agreements, requests were made due to agreement / contract deficiencies regarding various areas of reference which were stated are "the entire agreement between the parties related to the Available Programs" — (CPA Master Program Agreement, page 3 of 8, Section 6 Miscellaneous, 9e) Interpretation. This referred to four parts to the Master Agreement which were not fully disclosed.

September 25, 2017 @ 8:09 PM a request via email to Shana Doss as contact regarding the above mention agreements was made.

When reviewing the **CPA MASTER PROGRAM AGREEMENT**, Data Privacy & HIPAA BAA there were several areas which we need based on the reference of documentation and other agreements as part of the Master Program Agreement in the agreement executed on 4/18/2016.

2. Fees. Please provide fees and describe fees for **"CPA Package"** which Family Pharmacy is receiving services. Please provide the "Term Sheets" as described under ABDC's standard Master Agreement.

3. ABDC COMMITMENTS. Please provide the "Term Sheet for GNC Provider Network".

6. MISCELLANEOUS. (e) Interpretation. This describes the "Member Agreement", Credit Agreement and CPA Agreement as potentially separate agreements. (This paragraph states there are potentially four (4) parts to the master agreement including the Master Agreement). The statement these are the entire agreement between the parties related to Available Programs. Please provide these agreements or provide a statement as the CPA MASTER PROGRAM AGREEMENT is the entire agreement or, if the other agreements have not been received and signed off by Anywhere Pharmacy.

Please provide a statement to us so that we can document the existence or non existence of these agreements. These agreements potentially can provide insight to the issues at hand.

Reply from Corporate Executive Pharmacy: September 25, 2017 @ 8:56 pm.

"Unfortunately none of these items you mentioned below are available to us. After we consulted with our local attorneys early on they asked for these as well but CPA simple told me these are "agreements on file" and not shared with members."

These responses set a tone regarding the vendors to Anywhere Pharmacy as not responsive in the transparency in the agreements. The consulting firm to Anywhere Pharmacy should be the advocate and intermediary regarding the acquisition of the information requested. There was no correspondence forthcoming as a forward regarding the information requested.

The "CPA Package" is the agreement for the consulting firm which under the Master Agreement in Section 2. Fees states they have done the following and will continue to provide consulting with regard to the following as it is written in the agreement.

"2. FEES. CPA has negotiated special monthly pricing that replaces monthly fees in the Term Sheets for GNP Provider Network™; GNP-Link™ (pharmacy management, point-of-sale, and IVR systems and InSite from ABDC); Diabetes Shoppe®; THE Front End Solution (GNP promotions, first-to-shelf, planograms, zone pricing and merchandising); and Business Coaching (collectively, "CPA Package"). During the Term and for so long as Customer is a CPA Member, **Customer will pay such special pricing for the CPA Package, although some may require Customer to incur other expenses**, which are Customer's responsibility; provided however, if the parties replace this Master Agreement after the Term with ABDC.MPA.AGREEMENT.CPA.20100402 Page 2 of 8

ABDC's standard Master Agreement, **then-current monthly fees in the Term Sheets** will apply. Additional fees apply to Available Programs outside the CPA Package, and for transaction fees and optional program features selected by Customer such as promotional materials, newsletters and educational programs."

The above highlighted areas are just a few of the provisions within the agreements that provides no disclosure of the detail of the "Fees" and / or there is no disclosure or providing of the "Term Sheets". In the above as well there is no indication of what the costs / fees are for the "Available Programs outside the CPA Package", "transaction fees and optional program features" etcetera.

With non-disclosure of these fees / costs, Anywhere Pharmacy cannot know or budget for these expenses. Thus, charges can be made by CPA without basis for the actual costs / fees.

AB Drug Corporation referred to as (ABDC) in the CPA Master Program Agreement is the apparent PSAO for Anywhere Pharmacy. Section 4. Customer Commitments. This section refers to ABDC throughout this section and remainder of the agreement. The issue is there is no detail as to costs basis for the purchase, reimbursement, charts or excel spread sheets not reference to a web portal for the express basis of determining cost and reimbursement. There are no details only a "summarization" of what ABDC provides. There is No Transparency for ABDC and subsequent cost structure or reimbursement structure. They provide no means for determining how their DIR or Clawbacks are applied nor does the reference to the GNP Provider Network which provides access to PBM's.

Summary of ABDC / PSAO

It is important to have the PSAO Contract / Agreement / Documentation. This agreement will allow us to pinpoint and provide the detail needed in the final analytics. The full agreement will provide the answers to the questions below from the previous request. This agreement is something which FP should be provided as it is a part of full transparency as well as provides critical information needed by FP in measuring the cost and resulting profits in simple terms. By not having this agreement, FP is in a deficit on information / detail and language should any issues arise and litigation is needed. If the PSAO agreement is with AB Drug Corporation - they owe the contract / agreement documentation and any exhibits or reference agreements / contracts / documentation to FP for due diligence in exercising participation in the PSAO. Knowing what is signed and received is one thing. Agreements that refer to documentation as a reference and not received is of great concern such as the CPA Agreement. But, using a basis for the processing and cost of doing business with a PSAO and the underlying network and structure for FP is another. Without the proper documentation / agreement / Contract the question is - What do you know and do you have actionable knowledge should issues arise as they are now. Please be strong in your request for the PSAO Agreement / Contract / Documentation. Remember - **"You get exactly what you do not ask for"**. I look forward to your response and receiving the PSAO Agreement / Contract / Documentation.

Questions on PSAO / ABDC

These questions are normally answered in the actual PSAO Contract / Agreement. *We highly suggest the signed agreement be obtained by Anywhere Pharmacy regarding the PSAO.*

1 How much should you be reimbursed for the drugs you dispense?

    a What are the brand discounts?
    b What are the dispensing fees?
    c What are the MAC strategies and/or generic effective rate guarantees?
    d What are the contract provisions regarding copayments and usual and customary pricing?
    e What are the claw back and DIR provisions?

Even if we are only able to obtain rates from a few PBMs it will give us the opportunity to reconcile a defined number of claims.

2 How much do you pay for your prescription drugs?

    a Is your purchase price based on a pricing schedule? If so, please provide the most current version.
    b Is your cost based on WAC, AMP, ASP, or other sources? If so, what is the source and the cost multiplier?

Anything Anywhere Pharmacy can do to help us better understand the purchasing and sales pricing strategies will result in a better audit outcome.

The above were correspondence sent regarding the PSAO / ABDC Agreement. Answers were not provided based on any of the agreements at hand or provided based on requests. Should a dispute arise based on the agreements at hand from Anywhere Pharmacy a deficit in the defense of allegations brought will be apparent as there is apparently no basis for an objective defense.

An observation which needs to be pursued is the potential payments being received from the various vendors to CPA in addition to what Anywhere Pharmacy is paying for the advocacy of this vendor. This view is based on the fact they stated they negotiated the agreements in the CPA Master Program Agreement. Section 2. Fees "***CPA has negotiated special monthly pricing that replaces monthly fees*** in the Term Sheets for GNP Provider Network™; GNP-Link™ (pharmacy management, point-of-sale, and IVR systems and InSite from ABDC); Diabetes Shoppe®; THE Front End Solution (GNP promotions, first-to-shelf, planograms, zone pricing and merchandising); and Business Coaching (collectively, "CPA Package")."

A question arises from the above highlighted area as to what is the negotiated special monthly pricing that replaces the monthly fees. This information is not disclosed in any of the agreements received from Anywhere Pharmacy. Additionally, this raises another question regarding the monthly fees paid to Computer Company Rx on the System Agreement - *Is CPA receiving part of the monthly fees paid for support by Anywhere Pharmacy to Computer Company Rx?*

Computer CompanyRx System Agreement

This is the revised new agreement reviewed and orally discussed with Corporate Executive Pharmacy on areas of concern or issue. The first part of the agreement is a Business Associate Agreement and HIPAA. These agreements are standard and specific to Anywhere Pharmacy. In this agreement there is a provision which on the surface seems harmless but in reality provides a basis for Computer Company Rx to use the data and sell it. The following has bee extracted from the agreement.

"(ii) for data aggregation services, if to be provided by Business Associate for the health care operations of Covered Entity pursuant to any agreements between the Parties evidencing their business relationship. For purposes of this Agreement, data aggregation services means the combining of Protected

*Health Information by Business Associate with the Protected Health Information received by Business Associate in its capacity as a business associate of **another covered entity**, to permit data analyses that relate to the health care operations of the respective covered entities."*

The highlighted area brings the perception and probability that the information will be shared with "another covered entity" not Anywhere Pharmacy.

The following is extracted from the renewal agreement and the current agreement in force. This limits the right of Anywhere Pharmacy to receive compensation based on the following and specific to the highlighted areas.

B. THE ABOVE CONSTITUTES A LIMITED WARRANTY AND IS THE ONLY WARRANTY PROVIDED BY THE VENDOR. THE VENDOR MAKES AND THE CUSTOMER RECEIVES NO OTHER WARRANTIES, EXPRESS OR IMPLIED, WRITTEN OR ORAL, AND THE CUSTOMER ACKNOWLEDGES THAT NO WARRANTIES EXTEND BEYOND THE DESCRIPTIONS AS HEREIN PROVIDED. THERE IS EXPRESSLY EXCLUDED ALL WARRANTIES OF MERCHANTABILITY OR FOR FITNESS FOR A PARTICULAR PURPOSE AND NONINFRINGEMENT. *THE VENDOR SHALL NOT BE LIABLE FOR ANY INDIRECT, CONSEQUENTIAL, SPECIAL, EXEMPLARY OR INCIDENTAL DAMAGES (INCLUDING BUT NOT BEING LIMITED TO LOST PROFITS, LOST INCOME, INCREASED EXPENSE, LOSS OF GOOD WILL OR LABOR COSTS). FURTHER, LIABILITY OF THE VENDOR FROM ANY AND ALL LEGAL AND EQUITABLE CAUSES, OF EVERY KIND AND CHARACTER, SHALL IN THE AGGREGATE NOT EXCEED THE AMOUNTS PAID TO VENDOR BY THE CUSTOMER FOR USE OF THE SOFTWARE LICENSE (AND NOT THE EQUIPMENT) IN THE SIX (6) MONTHS PRECEDING THE EVENT WHICH GIVES RISE TO THE CLAIM.* NO *ACTION, REGARDLESS OF ITS NATURE,*

ORIGIN, OR FORM, ARISING OUT OF THIS AGREEMENT SHALL BE BROUGHT BY THE CUSTOMER AFTER ONE YEAR FROM THE DATE OF INITIAL INSTALLATION OF THE EQUIPMENT.

VII. EQUIPMENT WARRANTIES AND LIMITATIONS OF LIABILITY

A. ALL WARRANTIES RELATING TO EQUIPMENT SOLD OR RENTED TO THE CUSTOMER UNDER THIS AGREEMENT SHALL BE LIMITED TO THOSE WARRANTIES AS PROVIDED BY THE ORIGINAL EQUIPMENT MANUFACTURER, AND VENDOR ITSELF MAKES NO EXPRESS OR IMPLIED WARRANTY AS TO SAID EQUIPMENT. <u>IN NO EVENT SHALL VENDOR BE LIABLE FOR SPECIAL, INDIRECT, OR CONSEQUENTIAL DAMAGES (INCLUDING BUT NOT BEING LIMITED TO LOSS OF PROFITS, LOSS OF INCOME, INCREASED EXPENSE, EXPENSES RELATED TO RECOVERY OR RESTORATION OF LOST DATA, OR LOSS OF GOOD WILL) ARISING FROM OR RELATING TO THE EQUIPMENT SOLD OR RENTED TO THE CUSTOMER EVEN IF THE VENDOR HAS BEEN ADVISED OF THE POSSIBILITY OR FORESEEABILITY OF SUCH DAMAGES. FURTHER, LIABILITY OF THE VENDOR FROM ANY AND ALL CAUSES, WHETHER NEGLIGENCE, BREACH OF CONTRACT, WARRANTY OR OTHERWISE, SHALL IN THE AGGREGATE NOT EXCEED THE AMOUNTS PAID TO VENDOR FOR VENDOR HARDWARE IN THE SIX (6) MONTHS PRECEDING THE EVENT WHICH GIVES RISE TO THE CLAIM.</u> FURTHER, THE CUSTOMER AGREES THAT THE VENDOR WILL NOT BE LIABLE FOR ANY LOST PROFITS, NOR FOR ANY CLAIM OR DEMAND AGAINST THE CUSTOMER BY ANY OTHER PARTY. NO ACTION, REGARDLESS OF ITS NATURE, ORIGIN, OR FORM, ARISING OUT OF THIS AGREEMENT SHALL BE BROUGHT BY

THE CUSTOMER AFTER ONE YEAR FROM THE DATE OF INSTALLATION OF THE EQUIPMENT.

III. VENDOR-CREATED SOFTWARE AND CONFIDENTIALITY

A. In addition to the above, both Vendor and Customer have made and will continue throughout the term of this Agreement to make available to the other party confidential and proprietary materials and information ("Proprietary Information"). All material and information provided by one party to the other relating to the business, technology, policies, procedures, customers and forms of that party or any of its affiliates, including information previously divulged or delivered relating to the aforementioned subject matter is hereby designated as and considered to be Proprietary Information. Each party shall maintain the confidentiality of the other's Proprietary Information and will not disclose such Proprietary Information without the prior written consent of the other party. In addition, neither party shall use the other party's Proprietary Information except as contemplated herein. <u>It is understood that the obligations set forth above in this section do not apply to materials or information that (a) are already, or otherwise become, generally known by third parties as a result of no act or omission of the receiving party; (b) subsequent to disclosure hereunder are lawfully received from a third party having the right to disseminate the information without restriction on disclosure; (c) are generally furnished to others by the disclosing party without restriction on disclosure; (d) were already known by the receiving party prior to receiving them from the disclosing party and were not received from a third party in breach of that third party's obligations of confidentiality; (e) are provided to third parties in accordance with Article XV, Vendor</u>

<u>Data Use and REMS Programs; or (f) are independently developed by the receiving party without the use of Proprietary Information of</u>

the disclosing party. *In the event of a material breach in the terms and conditions of this Article by any party to this Agreement, then and in such event, the non-breaching party shall be entitled to seek immediate injunctive relief and, in addition, such other relief as may be provided in law and in equity.*

The above highlighted allows Computer Company Rx Agreement to provide and receive renumeration for data from Anywhere Pharmacy. From the above highlighted area and extract is brought out below to point out that three words allows for this — *"do not apply"* which are bolded in the extract below.

It is understood that the obligations set forth above in this section **do not apply** to materials or information that:

PBM Agreements

The various PBM Agreements were reviewed and found to not be transparent or provide the additional information needed to validate the allowed payments to Anywhere Pharmacy. Additionally, they did not expressly define the DIR / Clawback provisions and application of such. The CPA Thread looks to have an involvement with these agreements.

The following agreements received were not complete agreements for a PBM.

Caremark
Envision
ESI
Optimum Rx
Prime Therapeutics

Recommendations

1. Affidavit to CPA regarding the receipt of **any and all compensation** from any of the negotiated agreements with vendors which are contracted by Anywhere Pharmacy due to recommendation by CPA and contracts executed.
2. Request current agreement details and all agreements referenced by the Contracts signed.
3. To renegotiate the current contracts to get better pricing and full transparency of all the agreements / contracts.
4. Put out an RFP to vendors for reply so that Anywhere Pharmacy controls the agreements and transparency of the agreements. This will provide that the agreements be complete so there can be a basis for proper business decisions.

RESERVE

We reserve the right to change, modify or correct any and all comments or conclusions expressed in the written observations should we be given additional information that would warrant such actions.

F. Randall Childers, Jr., CFC, DABFE
Randall Childers Consulting
ACFEI - Certified Forensic Consultant
DABFE -Diplomate American Board Forensic Examiners
Forensic Specialty - Self Funded Health Plans
Licensed Employee Benefit Consultant

1099 Issue

The following is a summary regarding the issuance of 1099's for payments made by the plan to both vendors and providers. The Plan Sponsor asked that this information be reviewed and summarized. The following is a summary of the information. The detailed 1099's and Plan Sponsors name along with the Contracted Administrator have bee left out. The totality of the information was provided to the Investigative Unit of the U. S. Treasury with all supporting information.

As a practioner in Forensics the detail is very import as used only based on objective data. Cases are built with objective data and facts provided to those who will determine ther merits of moving forward or not on a issue at hand.

Issue: Contracted TPA processed 1099's with their Name, Address and TIN. The proper party is the one who's plan it is and the actual filer which is the Plan Sponsor not the contracted TPA.

Plan Sponsor - Is the company who has the self funded plan and is considered the fiduciary / owner / responsible party. The plan sponsor contracts with various vendors for the Plan on their behalf. The Plan Sponsor is the Payer as it is their plan, their bank account, their contributions, money, their expenses. The Contracted TPA (Third Party Administrator) has a service agreement with the Plan Sponsor for processing. The Contracted TPA is not the payer but only a processor on behalf of the Plan Sponsor for payment of claims, vendors and general processing.

Contracted TPA - The role of a good TPA is a vital component of the success of a health plan. With the proper choice of the TPA can make the experience very good. There is a difference in a TPA vs an ASO (Insurance Company) administrative services only agreement. In the ASO, one will find very little flexibility in the design and structure of the plan. They will normally use a "shelf" structure as this is an easy way for them to implement and administer the plan. With a TPA however, they are structured to take the direction of the Plan Sponsor for implementation, processing and administer the plan based on this architecture chosen by the Plan Sponsor. A contracted TPA will work with the plan sponsor and allow the various vendors chosen independently by the plan sponsor and coordinate with these vendors for processing.

The TPA with a self funded plan will work with the plan sponsor via an Administrative Service Agreement and has several tasks for implementation of the vendors chosen by the plan sponsor for processing by the contracted TPA for the Plan:

Consult and educate the employer and participants.
Adjudicate and process benefits / claims.
Provide billing and record keeping services.
Provide access to information / reports 24 / 7 on your plan via internet secure portal.
Processing for Stoploss coverage chosen by the **plan sponsor**.
Analyze and select the network chosen by the **plan sponsor**.
Process the Prescription Benefit Management Company (PBM) chosen by the plan sponsor.
Analyze and select the UR/PreCert/Case Management/Disease Management Company chosen by the plan sponsor.
Provide support and auxiliary services where possible and appropriate.

Process government filings, reports including 1099's on behalf of and for the Plan Sponsor

The TPA does not own the Plan or assets of the plan. Thus, they are not the Payer but only a processor for the benefit of the Plan Sponsor. All information and contracts are owned by the Plan Sponsor with their name, address, EIN - Not the TPA.

1099's are to be issued under the Plan Sponsors Name, Address and EIN. Per the instructions provided by the Internal Revenue Service on General Instructions for Certain Information Returns 2018 (page 13):

K. Filer's Name, Taxpayer Identification Number (TIN), and Address.

> The filer's name and TIN should be consistent with the name and TIN used on the filer's other tax returns. the name on the filer's paying agent or service bureau must **not** be used in place of the name of the filer.

Taking of expenses from one entity and applying to another entity is not permissible. Using 1099's to reduce tax liability on an entity who "stole" expenses from a legitimate entity is considered fraud and corruption. This could be Tax Evasion.

Contracted TPA administers / process for 160 plans and per their representatives did this with all 160 plans which encompasses approximately 17,000 employee participants.

Contracted TPA was questioned on their change of process from previous years and stated it was legal based on a 2006 Actuarial Opinion and an additional opinion of a law firm in 2017. Note: opinions are just that. The specific circumstances may have not been communicated to those providing an opinion. It is apparent that Contracted TPA did not explore the real authority regarding this issue on the 1099's (Internal Revenue Service) but relied on these opinion letters and 26

CFR 1.6041-1 which has been taken out of context and applied as Contracted TPA saw fit to support their actions.

TPA's typically will go to a convention such as HCAA, SIIA, SPBA and hear an idea from another TPA and will use that information due to the other TPA stating they are doing it and have been for years. Typically, these are implemented with out the proper due diligence required when providing Processing / Administrative services under a federal program ERISA.

Contracted Administrator Issue

with Stoploss Filing

The following is a case where the Contracted Administrator did not file with the Stoploss Carrier for an Aggregate Stoploss Reimbursement. The Plan Sponsor had Aggregate Accommodation as part of the Stoploss agreement and paid a pepm fee for this protection. The following report was completed and assistance provided to the Plan Sponsor in getting the Aggregate Reimbursement.

The forensic report utilized an analytical comparison of the data provided and the agreements provided on the vendor architecture of the plan. The vendors to the plan each provided a specific area of expertise in the function of the Plan Sponsor Health Benefit Plan. This plan is a self funded plan utilizing Stoploss insurance as a protection to the health benefit plan from a risk basis in protecting the cash flow due to large claims on both a specific and aggregate protection level.

This report is designed to show the findings of the health benefit plan forensic analysis. Forensic practice in Health Benefits remains completely objective in making an accurate determination of the facts involved and the presentation of the facts.

Vendor Analysis TPA (Third Party Administrator)

Background

The contracted administrator for the health plan was Contracted Administrator. Contracted Administrator was a licensed administrator with the Kentucky Department of Insurance. The office location was xxxxxx KY 40067. The corporate headquarters was xxxxxxxxxxx, West Des Moines, IA, 50266-1054. Phone (xxx) xxx-xxx President Owner. Contracted Administrator successor per announcement provided by Owner on June 25, 2010 per acquisition is XXX Insurance Group (XXX) based in Long Beach, CA. In the announcement, a rebranding on Contracted Administrator to XXX Benefits Administrators (TBA) as the new name. Per announcement, V.P is the head of XXX Insurance Group. XXX Benefit Administrators Corporate office is listed as xxxxxxx, West Des Moines, IA, 50266-1054. Phone (xxx) xxx-xxxx per web portal abcdefg.com.

Contracted Administrator entered into an agreement with Plan Sponsor as the contracted administrator for the Plan Sponsor Health Benefit Plan on December 18, 2008 for an effective date starting January 1, 2009 per Administrative Service Agreement **(TAB 3 / Administrative Service Agreement)**. This agreement laid out the responsibilities of each party for the Plan Sponsor Health Benefit System. A Plan Document was produced by Contracted Administrator which listed the parameters of how the plan was to function. Trustees listed in the Plan Document were: HR Director, Human Resource Director; Kim Adair, Executive Director and Chip Cox, Chairman of the Board.

The following are the forensic findings on Plan Sponsor Health Benefit Plan.

A recreation of the plan year was done which included a full accounting per reports provided by Plan Sponsor from check registers, Bank Statements, reports from Contracted Administrator, reports from

AmeriScript (HealthSmart Rx), PBM Auditing Company and Spectrum Underwriting Managers. This information was compiled and entered into Quick Books. This provided a basis for a comparative analysis for each component of the plan. A full reconciliation of the US Bank Account was completed for utilization in the comparative analysis with a detailed Profit and Loss Statement and detailed Balance Sheet. **(See TAB 2, Profit and Loss, Balance Sheet and Reconciliation Reports)**.

Total administrative and other fees (see Fiduciary Request TAB 4) paid to Contracted Administrator for the 2009 Plan Year: $9,684.50 **(TAB 2, Profit and Loss, Professional Fees, Medical Administration Fees)**.

Accounting - (TAB 2)

Accounting for Plan Sponsor Health Benefit Account for the Plan Year 2009. The following results were found.

Medical Claims Category shows $106,632.92 which matches the Aggregate Reporting. **(TAB 2, Profit and Loss, Medical Claims)**

Prescription Claims Category shows $25,214.29 which matches the Aggregate Reporting. **(TAB 2, Profit and Loss, Prescription Claims)**

There were three checks written as reimbursements under the category of Flexible Reimbursement Account which total $169.02. These checks appear to have been written to reimburse medical expenses and applied to the Health Benefit Plan Account. If these expenses were actual medical claim expenses they should have been calculated in the Medical Claims Category which would have increased this category to by $169.02 and should have been reimbursed as part of the aggregate filing. Since this is an unknown fact, this amount should be transferred to the Health Benefit Account from the Flexible Reimbursement account to make the Health Benefit Account whole.

Additionally, there were reimbursements received from Spectrum / Zurich which do not show up on the January 2009 through December

2009 accounting as these were received in 2010. In addition, Rebates were received for the 2009 Plan year from AmeriScript/HealthSmart which are to be applied to the 2009 Plan Year and reimbursement from the Flexible Reimbursement Account. Thus, the account balance after applying these amounts would be:

Category	Amount	Received
Balance as of 12/31/2009	-$15,784.85	
Specific Reimbursement	$7,562.45	01/02/2010
Specific Reimbursement	$7,172.12	01/28/2010
Aggregate Reimbursement	$20,704.94	03/02/2010
Rx Rebates 2009	$807.00	10/14/2010
Flexible Reimbursement Account	$169.02	1/22/09 and 2/26/09
Total	$20,630.68	

There are three checks that have not cleared as of 02/18/2013 from reconciliation through the period. Ck# 1144 $288.00 to Randall Childers, Ck# 1163 $85.00 and Ck# 1173 $143.65 to Dallas Medical PLLC. These amounts are outstanding and still due from the Plan Sponsor Health Benefit Account.

In view of the balance as stated above, Plan Sponsor could be reimbursed for the amounts deposited above the required contributions from the plan. The additional contributions to the plan were:

Category	Amount	Date
Account Opening	$100.00	1/15/2009
Additional Deposit	$5,000.00	07/01/2009
Additional Deposit	$15,500.00	12/30/2009
Total	$20,600.00	

This reimbursement would leave a $30.68 balance for the plan year. This transaction would make whole Plan Sponsor.

Stoploss

The agreement with Spectrum Underwriters and Zurich for the Stoploss protection of the Plan Sponsor Health Plan for the aggregate coverage included a provision for Aggregate Accommodation which has been validated per the agreement provided by Spectrum Underwriters. This provision is designed to protect the cash flow of the plan in the event it exceeds the attachment point either by contracted amount or actual which ever is greater.

The contracted administrator Contracted Administrator has an obligation for timely filings and processing per the Administrative Service Agreement signed on December 18, 2008 for an effective agreement of January 1, 2009 by Kim Adair, Executive Director of Plan Sponsor.

In Section 3.18 the TPA (Third Party Administrator) agreed to the following: (TAB 3, Administrative Agreement, page 8, 3.18)

3.18 Notify the excess loss insurance company of any potential large Claims which may become a Claim under the excess loss coverage.

On behalf of the Plan, the TPA will file in a timely manner any Claims for benefits under the excess loss policies.

Promptly forward to the Plan Sponsor any premium and other notices received from the excess loss insurance company concerning the policy.

The Plan Sponsor Health Benefit Plan Stoploss agreement included Aggregate Accommodation. This amount was charged to Plan Sponsor and paid at $1.00 per participant per month for a total of $301.00 for the 2009 Plan Year.

The Monthly Aggregate Accommodation Endorsement (Zurich American Insurance Company) states: (TAB 5, Stoploss Policy, Monthly Aggregate Accommodation Endorsement)

After the end of the fourth (4th) month that this policy has been in force and through the (11th) month, the Company will advance to and pay to the Policyholder as a loan the Aggregate Stoploss reimbursement, if any, within ten (10) days after the Company's acceptance of the Proof of Loss and verification that Eligible Plan Benefits have been incurred and Paid within the Benefit Period as shown in the SCHEDULE OF Stoploss INSURANCE.

Summary of findings: The Aggregate Claim was filed on January 7, 2010 to Spectrum Underwriting Managers, Inc. By Contracted Administrator. The Aggregate Claim was paid by Spectrum Underwriting Managers, Inc. on February 15, 2010 check number 1370157402 in the amount of **$20,704.94**.

The aggregate claims for the Plan Sponsor exceeded the attachment point starting in June 2009 the sixth (6th) month of the plan. This amount in June 2009 was $3,657.97 in excess of the attachment point. This increased each month of the 2009 plan year to a total of $20,704.94.

The timely filings of these claims were *not* done by Contracted Administrator as stated in 3.18 of the Administrative Service Agreement. This created a **breach** of the Administrative Agreement signed on December 18, 2008 for an effective date of January 1, 2009. The breach **created a financial hardship** on the Plan Sponsor Health Benefit Plan and caused Plan Sponsor to additionally fund **$20,500** to the plan in excess of the contracted amounts. On July 2009 Plan Sponsor funded **$5,000** and an additional **$15,500** in December 2009. The timely filings of the excess of the Aggregate Attachment Point by Contracted Administrator would have prevented this hardship. (TAB 2, Profit and Loss, Health Plan Deposits)

Based on this information and the following objective data, Plan Sponsor should request from Contracted Administrator the following due to breach of Administrative Agreement.

Aggregate Accommodation fees paid Plan Year 2009: $301.00

. filings from Contracted Administrator. Contracted Administrator was not timely in submission of the Aggregate Claims for Plan Sponsor Health Benefit Plan. This is shown in the following analysis on total reimbursements received from Spectrum / Zurich.

		Spectrum Specific and Aggregate Reimbursements PS 2009 Plan Year				
Type	Who	Amount	Date	Check #	PS Deposit Date	Aggregating Total
Specific	Owens	$26,851.71	08/14/09	1370149458	09/01/09	$26,851.71
Specific	Owens	$295.35	09/08/09	1370150513	09/17/09	$27,147.06
Specific	Enos	$1,369.91	10/14/09	1370152128	10/22/09	$28,516.97
Specific	Owens	$3,850.07	10/14/09	1370152128	10/22/09	$32,367.04
Specific	Scott	$4,730.01	11/02/09	1370152928	11/10/09	$37,097.05
Specific	Scott	$158.18	11/12/09	1370153322	11/25/09	$37,255.23
Specific	Owens	$570.42	11/23/09	1370153651	12/03/09	$37,825.65
Specific	Scott	$509.43	12/24/09	1370154988	01/05/10	$38,335.08
Specific	Enos	$1,184.28	12/24/09	1370154990	01/05/10	$39,519.36
Specific	Enos	$5,094.99	12/24/09	1370154990	01/05/10	$44,614.35
Specific	Owens	$773.75	12/28/09	1370155112	01/05/10	$45,388.10
Specific	Enos	$1,013.51	01/19/10	1370153075	01/28/10	$46,401.61
Specific	Owens	$6,044.05	01/19/10	1370156073	01/28/10	$52,445.66
Specific	Scott	$114.56	01/19/10	1370156076	01/28/10	$52,560.22
Aggregate	2009 Plan	$20,704.94	02/15/10	1370157402	03/02/10	$73,265.16
		$73,265.16				

PBM Auditing

Plan Sponsor Health Benefit Plan entered into an agreement with PBM Auditing Company and Contracted Administrator for PBM Prospective based auditing on December 18, 2008 for an effective date of January 1, 2009. **(TAB 7, PBMA Documentation)**

The following is a comparative analysis to establish the audited amounts and subsequent payments for this service were done and processed by Contracted Administrator.

The Plan Sponsor Health Benefit Plan was billed by PBM Auditing Company and submitted to Contracted Administrator for payment from the Plan Sponsor Health Plan Account. The amounts paid by the Plan Sponsor Health Benefit Plan were $206.50. **(TAB 2, Profit and Loss, Professional Fees, PBM Auditing Fees)**

The analysis shows the amount of reductions per the prospective audit were not applied by Contracted Administrator for a net payment to the PBM AmeriScript. Thus, a breach of agreement occurred on behalf of Contracted Administrator. From analysis of the AmeriScript Billing and the amounts processed by Contracted Administrator shows the audited PBM Billings completed by PBM Auditing Company and submitted to Contracted Administrator was not done.

The Aggregate Report, Billing Reports from AmeriScript and the audited amounts from PBM Auditing Company were completed on a comparative analysis. That analysis and confirmation of the various reports shows no audited reductions were processed by Contracted Administrator.

Auditing Fees charged to the Plan:	**$ 206.50**
Non processed Audit findings:	**$ 227.36**
Total of Findings:	**$ 433.86**

Note: The probability exists on non accurate filing of specific and aggregate claims by Contracted Administrator which has a significance of possible *insurance fraud* for non application of audited amounts to the specific and aggregate filings with Spectrum Underwriters / Zurich.

Fiduciary Request - (TAB 4)

On August 24, 2009 a request from HR Director, Trustee was sent to Contracted Administrator requesting compensation be paid to F. Randall Childers, Jr., as Agent and Consultant of Record. This is a Fiduciary request to the Contracted Administrator Contracted Administrator.

Reviewing the check registers and payments to the various entities as professional fees it was found the directive sent to Contracted Administrator was not followed. Fact, Contracted Administrator paid themselves the fees instead of paying based on the directive of the Trustee. This is a **breach agreement and a high probability of theft**.

The following information shows the results of these finding from the analysis and processing of the check registers supplied by Contracted Administrator and reconciled against the US Bank Statements for the Plan Sponsor Health Benefit Plan. The Fiduciary Request was sent via U.S. Mail, Fax and Emailed to Contracted Administrator.

The requested amounts are due to breach of agreement and not adhering to the directive of the Trustee for the Plan Sponsor Health Benefit Plan.

Fees retained by Contracted Administrator and not abiding by Fiduciary Request.

Fees 9/1/2009 to 12/31/2009: $1,260.00

PBM AmeriScript (HealthSmart Rx) (TAB 6)

A comparative Analysis of the PBM reporting and billing to Contracted Administrator processing and payment of the billing shows significance in findings. The following chart shows the billings by month from AmeriScript and the processing by Contracted Administrator.

| AmeriScript / HealthSmart Monthly Billing vs AA processing ||||
2009	Rx Claims Billed	AA Processed	Difference
January	$1,374.76		$1,374.76
February	$2,604.66	$1,374.76	$1,229.90
March	$2,436.91	$2,604.66	-$167.75
April	$2,108.36		$2,108.36
May	$2,034.43	$5,460.06	-$3,425.63
June	$2,613.70	$1,119.64	$1,494.06
July	$1,844.07	$2,613.70	-$769.63
August	$2,979.13	$1,009.20	$1,969.93
September	$1,962.32	$3,814.00	-$1,851.68
October	$1,694.41	$1,962.32	-$267.91
November	$2,198.54	$1,694.41	$504.13
December	$1,975.80	$3,561.54	-$1,585.74
Total	$25,827.09	$25,214.29	$612.80

Based on the data received from HealthSmart Rx (AmeriScript) and Contracted Administrator reporting, there was a lag in processing the Prescription claims by as much as 60 days for the period January through May from the Contracted Administrator. The balance of the months appeared to have a 15 to 30 day lag.

Per HealthSmart Rx, claims were sent via electronic (EDI) and US Mail for processing. Electronic submission was done same day or next day.

In the comparison of the information, the actual billing for Rx (Prescriptions) vs the Contracted Administrator processed billing established a $612.80 difference. This additional amount of claims was not included in the Aggregate Filing with Spectrum. The $612.80 was the billing for 12/31/2009.

This analysis also confirms the audited PBM claims were not processed by Contracted Administrator due to the match of the gross bill from Ameriscript to the processed payments by Contracted Administrator.

In addition, the probability exists for an earlier filing for the Aggregate reimbursements from Spectrum / Zurich should have been done in the fifth month of the plan had Contracted Administrator processed the prescription claims as received in the billings from Ameriscript timely.

The following is a letter sent to the Contracted Administrator after all objective findings were reviewed. The result was the Contracted Administrator complied with the request.

PRIVILEGED AND CONFIDENTIAL SETTLEMENT

COMMUNICATION REULE 408

RESPONSE

Wednesday, October 9, 2013

Allegation: failure to timely file aggregate claims

Contracted Administrator agreement with Plan Sponsor required Contracted Administrator to file timely.

Section 3.18 in the Administrative Service Agreement states:

3.18 Notify the excess loss insurance company of any potential large Claims which may become a Claim under the excess loss coverage.
*On behalf of the Plan, the TPA will file in a **timely manner** any Claims for benefits **under the excess loss policies**.*
Promptly forward to the Plan Sponsor any premium and other notices received from the excess loss insurance company concerning the policy.

The Stoploss Agreement with Spectrum Underwriters / Zurich American Insurance included Aggregate Accommodation and Specific Advancement in the policy for protection of the plan and its assets. This protection required timely filings by Contracted Administrator and the Contracted Administrator to file these claims after the 4th month that the policy has been in force. **(Monthly Aggregate Accommodation Endorsement Zurich American Insurance Company)**

Allegation: PBM audit fees not earned

Contracted Administrator agreement with Plan Sponsor required Contracted Administrator to process the audited amounts per the Administrative Service Agreement. It is clear that Contracted Administrator did not fulfill this obligation. It is immaterial the amount that was or was not processed. The fact is Contracted Administrator neglected whether intentionally or non intentionally to process this area for the audited PBM Claims. The failure to process by Contracted Administrator resulted in cost and lost audited savings to the plan. There is no offset between the fees and the audited results.

Allegation: Contracted Administrator failed to comply with a fiduciary request

The fiduciary request by the plan trustee required these fees be paid to Broker for Plan Sponsor. The terminology in the Administrative Service Agreement Fee Schedule stated: ***Broker fee of $10.00 per covered Employee per month.*** The Plan and Trustees have the authority to state who their Broker is and to direct that payment accordingly. This is not at the discretion of Contracted Administrator as they are the Contracted Administrator.

Allegation: Improper payment from Health Benefit Plan Account

Contracted Administrator agreement with Plan Sponsor required Contracted Administrator to process the claims properly per the Administrative Service Agreement.

The drafter of the Forensic Report is not available to Contracted Administrator.

Contracted Administrator will be at their own expense in auditing their own administrative services and processing.

Based on the above and for the reasons previously stated Plan Sponsor holds to their original request.

In summary, the vendors to the plan performed as contracted with the exception of Contracted Administrator. The findings are significant for the probability of breach of agreements, fraud and theft. This report was compiled from information obtained in written format and verbal.

I reserve the right to change, modify or correct any and all comments or conclusions expressed in my written observations should I be given additional information that would warrant such actions.

F. Randall Childers, Jr., CFC, DABFE
Certified Forensic Consultant
Diplomate American Board of Forensic Examiners

Acronyms Used in this Book

ABC - Agent, Broker, Consultant
ASO - Administrative Services Only
AWP - Average Wholesale Price
BAA - Business Associate Agreement
CA - Contracted Administrator
CLASS Act - Community Living Assistance Services and Support Act
CM - Case Management
COBRA - Consolidated Omnibus Budget Reconciliation Act
DM - Disease Management
DOI - Department of Insurance
EIN - Employer Identification Number
E&O - Errors and Omission
FSA - Flexible Spending Accounts
HITECH - Health Information Technology for Economic and Clinical Health Act
IBNR - Incurred But Not Received
IRBNP - Incurred Received But Not Processed
MAC - Maximum Allowable Cost
MC - Managed Care
MGU - Managing General Underwriter
NDC - National Drug Code
Non PAR - Not Participating
NPI - National Provider Identifier
NPN - National Producer Number

OON - Out of Network
PAR - Participating
PBM - Prescription Benefit Manager
PEPM - Per Employee Per Month
PHI - Protected Health Information
PMPM - Per Member Per Month
PPACA - Patient Protection and Affordable Care Act
PPO - Preferred Provider Organization
PreCert -Pre Certification
PS - Plan Spnosor
TPA - Third Party Administrator
UCR - Usual Customary and Reasonable
UR - Utilization Review
URAC - Utilization Review Accreditation Commission

Bibliography

Busch, Rebecca Saltiel. *Healthcare Fraud: Auditing and Detection Guide.* John Wiley & Sons, 2012.

Cohen, Martin. *Critical Thinking Skills for Dummies.* John Wiley & Sons, 2015.

DeScherer, Dorinda D., and Terence M. Meyers. *Employee Benefits Answer Book.* 8th ed. New York: Aspen, 2003. Print.

Garner, John C. *Health Insurance Answer Book.* 7th ed. New York: Aspen, 2006. Print.

Harker, Carlton. *Self-funding of Health Care Benefits.* Ed. Mary E. Brennan. 4th ed. Brookfield, WI: International Foundation of Employee Benefit Plans, 1998. Print.

Internal Revenue Service. Web. 05 July 2011. <http://WWW.irs.gov>. Kentucky Office of Insurance. *Insurance Laws & Regulations.* 2006 Ed., Frankfort: Thompson/West, 2007. Print.

Madinger, John. *Money laundering: a guide for criminal investigators --* 3rd ed. p.cm.

Morris, Robyn C. *Flexible Benefits Answer Book.* 4th ed. New York: Aspen, 2003. Print.

Peck, Esq., Ron E. "TPA Fiduciary Duties' in Light of Recent New Jersey Case Law." *MyHealthGuide Newsletter for the Self funded Community* (15 Apr. 2010). *MyHealthGuide.com*. 15 Apr. 2010. Web. 16 Apr. 2010. <http://www.myhealthguide.com/>.

Pedneault, Stephen. Fraud 101: *Techniques and Strategies for Understanding Fraud*, 3rd Edition. John Wiley & Sons, 2009.

Russo, Esq., Adam V. "Mind the Gap' - Don't Get Stuck With a Bill Your Stoploss Insurer Excludes." *MyHealthGuide Newsletter for the Self funded Community* (21 Nov. 2010). *MyHealthGuide.com*. 21 Nov. 2010. Web. 22 Nov. 2010. <http://www.myhealthguide.com/>.

The U.S. Department of Labor Home Page. Web. 05 July 2011. <http://www.dol.gov>.

Trachtman, Joel P. *The Tools of Argument: How the Best Lawyers Think, Argue and Win*. CreateSpace Independent Publishing Platform, 2013.